GETTING
THIN

By Gabe Mirkin, M.D., and Marshall Hoffman:

THE SPORTSMEDICINE BOOK

GETTING
THIN

All about Fat—
How You Get It, How You Lose It,
How You Keep It off for Good

GABE MIRKIN, M.D.
WITH LAURA FOREMAN

Little, Brown and Company
Boston–Toronto–London

FIRST PAPERBACK EDITION

LIBRARY OF CONGRESS CATALOGING IN PUBLICATION DATA

Mirkin, Gabe.
  Getting thin.

  Includes index
  1. Reducing diets. 2. Obesity. I. Title
RM222.2.M54   1983   613.2'5   82-25895
ISBN 0-316-57439-2

Our special thanks to dieticians Terry Heller, R.D., and Althea Zanecosky, R.D., as well as to Susan Sandler, Ph.D., for their valuable assistance.

Thanks most of all to our editors, Genevieve Young and Dona Munker, who have bled, suffered, anguished, and been the driving force for this book.

10   9   8   7

MV PA
Designed by Susan Windheim

Published simultaneously in Canada
by Little, Brown & Company (Canada) Limited

PRINTED IN THE UNITED STATES OF AMERICA

To Mona, my love and inspiration

AUTHOR'S NOTE

Before embarking on any diet or exercise program, including those suggested in this book, it is a good idea to check with your physician to see if you have any condition that might be aggravated by a reducing diet or strenuous exercise.

CONTENTS

Morale · Excuses, Excuses · Substituting Activity for Food ·
Family and Peer Pressures · Calorie Counting · Relaxation
· Joining Up · The New You

Other Methods · Acupuncture · Jaw Wiring · Hypnosis · Negative Biofeedback · Hope for the Future? · Antibsorptives · Stomach Ballooning · The Last Word

What Have You Learned? · Where Do You Go from Here? · Backsliding · Getting to Know Your "New Self" · Tomorrow and Forever

GETTING
THIN

1.

MYTHS ABOUT FAT

Anyone who tells you that being fat is a simple problem with a simple solution is either lying or badly misinformed.

The same goes for anyone who says that all you need to be thin for life is a little gumption and a strict diet.

Yet there are millions of people who believe both these propositions, along with a lot more misinformation, quasi-facts, semitruths, and just plain nonsense that surround the subject of fat.

An estimated 80 million Americans are overweight. Fifteen percent of all Americans under the age of thirty are too fat, and the incidence of obesity in people over thirty rises to 30 percent.

The fat among us are spending a lot of money trying to get slim. They enrich the coffers of the weight-loss industry to the tune of some $10 billion a year. Among other things, the money goes for diet pills, diet books, doctors' fees, spas and health clubs, weight-reduction centers, reducing equipment, diet foods and beverages, and a variety of gimmicks that can't possibly reduce anything but your bank account.

WHAT YOU DON'T KNOW CAN HURT YOU

The extent to which the nonsense is believed indicates the extent of today's passion for slimness. Americans are in a frenzy to be thin, and they seem willing to try almost anything to get that way. People who are ordinarily sane and sensible can turn totally irrational when it comes to losing weight. They're willing to try the most bizarre gimmicks and believe the most outlandish promises in their quest for slenderness.

Many have found out by now that the gimmicks are useless and the promises hollow. There are no easy answers. If you're still looking for one, you're reading the wrong book.

What this book will give you is the truth. Yes, it's possible to get thin and stay that way. But it's hardly simple and it's seldom easy. Fat is a tough and complicated enemy. If you hope to beat it, you have to understand it. Knowledge — not weird gizmos and "miracle" diets — is your best ally.

How do you know if you're fat? Why and how do you get fat? How does your body tend to keep you fat once you get that way? What does your body do with the food you eat? Is overeating really your problem? Or is something wrong with your lifestyle? Are fat people and thin people constitutionally different in some way?

These are a few of the basic questions you have to be able to answer if you're going to win the war with fat.

Most chronic dieters are disciplined and determined people who've tried long and hard to lose weight and keep it off. They may have shed pounds successfully many times, only to watch them creep back into place. They start running out of patience and running out of hope.

If you're one of these people, don't quit yet. You may have been losing the battle because you weren't armed with the facts. Learn them. Then rethink your strategy and tactics. You'll find that your chances of being slender for life are much improved.

MYTH VS. FACT

Begin by forgetting some of the things you think you know. Consider these common myths about fat:

1. *Fat is ugly.*

This may be true here and now, but not always and everywhere. The "fat is ugly" value judgment arose in America only about sixty years ago. Before that, well-fleshed women were considered beautiful, and stout men were considered prosperous-looking. Historically speaking, fat was beautiful for thousands of years. There are many parts of the world where it still is today.

2. *Fat is unhealthy.*

It depends on how you look at it. It's true that being too fat is bad for your health. But the ability to store *some* fat is vital to your very life. Fat is a highly convenient and portable source of necessary water, energy, and heat. Human beings need it to procreate. And, in a pinch, it can even keep your brain from starving. Mankind would never have survived as a species without the ability to store fat. And over the course of evolution, being fat upped the odds for an individual to live to a ripe old age.

3. *Fat people get that way because they eat too much.*

Some do, but many don't. The most common cause of obesity is underactivity, not overeating. Strange as it seems, people who're sedentary and overweight usually eat less than people who're slim and active.

4. *Your glands make you fat.*

Hardly ever. It's true that the hormones your glands produce play a role in whether you're fat or thin. But you don't get fat because your glands malfunction. You make them malfunction by being fat.

5. *If your parents are fat, you're fated to be fat.*

Having fat parents can stack the deck against you. So can allowing yourself to remain overweight into the later years of childhood and adolescence. But you're never doomed to be fat for life, either by your genes or your upbringing.

6. *People get fat because they have emotional problems.*

Not true. Research indicates overwhelmingly that fat people are no weaker emotionally, or less stable psychologically, than thin ones. Yes, fat people may overeat in times of emotional stress. So do many thin ones. Being "unhappy" isn't why people become overweight. However, many people are unhappy *because* they're overweight — and with good reason. Fat people are the targets of irrational prejudice in the United States.

7. *If you want to be thin, you have to diet.*

Restricting your calorie intake is certainly helpful if you're trying to lose weight. But diet is not the true key to weight control. No serious scientist still believes that diet alone can make the average person permanently slim. In separate landmark studies, two eminent obesity experts, Dr. Albert Stunkard of the University of Pennsylvania and Dr. Alvin Feinstein of Yale, showed that the overwhelming majority of people who successfully lose weight through dieting quickly regain their lost weight. To lose weight and keep it off, most overweight people need a program that also includes behavior modification and exercise. Claims to the contrary by the never-ending stream of diet gurus fly in the face of solid scientific fact.

Exercise is the key. Weight loss through diet alone is ultimately useless for the vast majority of dieters. If you lose weight this way, your chances of keeping it off for five years are one in a hundred. The "diet only" approach is also dangerous. It sets you up for the "yo-yo syndrome" of loss and gain that can shorten your life.

8. *Snacking makes you fat.*

On the contrary. Snacking on healthful, low-calorie foods can help make you thin. Frequent, small meals are much less fattening than infrequent, large ones. Nibblers stay thin; gorgers get fat.

9. *Exercise doesn't count in weight loss. After all, you have to walk for seventeen hours to lose a single pound.*

This is the most misleading myth of all. Regular exercise doesn't just burn more calories while you're doing it. It gears your body to burn additional calories around the clock, even while you sleep. In addition, exercise is the only method proved effective in altering your appetite permanently. Moderate exercise doesn't make you hungrier. It makes you eat less.

10. *Weight loss alone won't get rid of "cellulite"—clogged tissue that causes skin to dimple on especially fat parts of your body.*

Rest assured you don't have a cellulite problem. There's no such thing as cellulite. Fat is fat is fat. Dimpling is caused by fat pushing up between tiny ligaments that run from the skin's surface through the fat layer to the muscles underneath. When the fat goes, the dimples go. You won't get rid of them by using any special pill, food, exercise, or massage technique.

11. *You can "spot-reduce" a pot belly or flabby bottom by exercising the muscles in those areas.*

Spot reduction is a fiction. You may be able to tighten up muscles selectively, but this won't affect the overlay of fat. Sit-ups won't make your belly disappear, and rolling around on your rear won't flatten it. When you lose fat, you lose it from wherever it was deposited in the first place. Look at tennis players. They spend hours every day exercising only one arm. Yet both arms are equal in fat content.

12. *Heat belts, rubber exercise suits, body wraps, and saunas will melt off unwanted fat.*

All they'll reduce is your bank book. These devices all work on the same principle. Heating an area will cause cells in that area to lose water and become dehydrated. The fluid loss will give you a loss in inches—

for just as long as it takes you to drink a glass of water. When you do, the fluid returns immediately to the places it's needed, and the inches come right back.

YOU'RE ON YOUR WAY

If these facts challenge some of your long-held notions about fat, be encouraged. You're on the road toward rethinking your weight problem and dealing with it realistically.

Up until now, bad information may have handicapped your best efforts to lose weight. But once you junk the myths and learn the facts, you'll find that past disappointments need not repeat themselves.

Man is probably the most physically inactive mammal on earth. He is also one of the fattest. A study published in *Nature* magazine showed that of forty-nine mammals surveyed, man was one of the five fattest. We are literally fatter than pigs, for instance. The study related body-fat percentages to physical activity levels, finding that the animals that move least accumulate the most fat.

It's also a fact that there's no such thing as a fat sponge or a fat oyster. Creatures that don't move at all cannot store fat.

2.

IS FAT UGLY?

Look at the pages of *Vogue* or *Glamour*, and an angular Aphrodite stares out at you.

Her eyes look huge in her famished face. Her cheekbones jut out over cavernous hollows. Ribs outline her breastless torso, and her hips are as straight and flat as two-by-fours.

This whip-thin image looks less like a woman than like an adolescent boy. But in America today, she's the epitome of high fashion and sensual allure. Women gaze on her with envy, men with admiration and lust.

CHANGING TIMES, CHANGING TASTES

Our modern bias for slimness is so strong that you might think thinness has always been worshiped. In fact, nothing could be further from the truth.

As aesthetics go, the skinny Venus is quite new on the scene, and her popularity is by no means universal. As a symbol of beauty, she's the exception, not the rule — both historically and geographically. She would have horrified our own ancestors, who liked their women lush. And she would be equally unappetizing to the average Egyptian or Eskimo, even today.

And what of Adonis, the ideal of male attractiveness? Today, it's the lean and lanky man whom we mentally link with sexy women, expensive cars, executive suites, and all-around high living. But not so long ago, a "fine figure of a man" was also a rather fat figure. Stoutness was associated with power, virility, and success.

I mention men here only in passing. As you'll see in Chapter 9, obesity is far more a female problem than a male one. To begin with, women tend naturally to be fatter than men. And while men are often concerned with the health problems obesity poses, women worry far more about how excess fat affects their looks.

So for women especially, it's useful to bring some perspective to the cosmetic considerations of being overweight by modern standards. The point to remember is this: what's "ugly" and what's "beautiful" are matters of taste, and tastes are shaped by the culture one lives in. Thin may be "in" here and now. But in a longer and wider view, fat is the easy winner as the prevailing standard of beauty.

The Voluptuous Venus

One of the earliest surviving tributes to female beauty is a little statuette called the Venus of Willendorf. This lady dates back at least 20,000 years

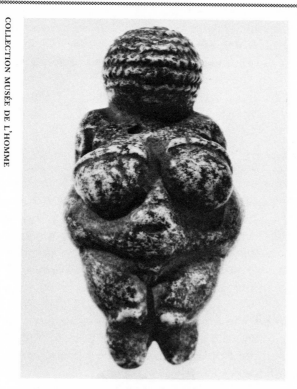

COLLECTION MUSÉE DE L'HOMME

The Venus of Willendorf

to a time when men were hunting reindeer for a living and depending on caves to keep out a year-round chill.

In form, she looks a lot like a double-dip ice cream cone. She is, by any standard, enormously fat. But in her day, she was thought to be as gorgeous as she was globular. She was, quite literally, a lot of woman.

Beauty and Body Types

As scientists would put it, women are natural endomorphs. An "endomorph" is a person who tends to be soft and round. The other two body types generally cited nowadays are "mesomorphs" and "ectomorphs." Mesomorphs are muscular and athletic, and ectomorphs are long-limbed and lean. Women are drastically underrepresented in the two thinner categories.

"Till early in this century, Venus was almost always drawn in the guise of an endomorph; moon-faced, pear-shaped and well fleshed out." So concludes anthropologist Anne Scott Beller in her fascinating book *Fat and Thin: A Natural History of Obesity*. She notes that only in the last sixty or seventy years did fat fade as the hallmark of feminine appeal.

The Willendorf Venus, essence of endomorphy, was but the first and largest in a long line of big beauties who filled the fantasies of their contemporaries.

Beauty through the Ages

The fertility goddesses of early primitive cultures were usually heavy-breasted and ripely rotund, with bulging bellies and sturdy thighs. While far more graceful, the classical goddesses of Greece and Rome were no lightweights either. As portrayed in statuary, they were, well, statuesque.

Hera, queen of the gods, was often depicted as regally stout. The immortal Venus de Milo was hardly a size six. Nor was the Venus Callipyge, who gave us the word *callipygian*, meaning "having a sumptuous rear."

Even heftier were the broad-beamed Renaissance beauties of Titian and Giorgione, followed by the enormous nudes of Rubens and the buxom matrons of the Impressionists. All these and many more testify to a taste through the ages for fleshy women.

You see it in popular illustration as well as fine art as you move toward modern times. Look through any early Sears, Roebuck catalogue. Tightly corseted models of hourglass perfection abound.

Some Fabulous Fatties

History offers us some chubby real-life heroines. Cleopatra is a timeless sex symbol whose charm brought emperors and empires to their knees. Yet some accounts tell us that the Queen of the Nile, though short, weighed in at about 150 pounds.

The brilliant and stormy Catherine the Great of Russia, a renowned beauty, grew quite stout in her later years. Yet she remained one of the most pursued (and caught) women in history. She wore out an awesome string of lovers, and she was still happily cavorting with the last of them when she died at the age of sixty-seven.

The world's reigning beauty toward the end of the nineteenth-century was Lillie Langtry, first official mistress of the future King Edward VII of England. Lillie was much sought after by artists as a model, and by kings and princes for her other services. But when Pears Soap offered to pay her weight in pounds sterling for an endorsement, the company had to fork over 134 pounds. Given her moderate height, Lillie would have fared badly on most of today's height-weight charts.

So would her American contemporary, actress Lillian Russell. Miss Russell's numerous admirers included the fabulously rich Diamond Jim Brady. Known for her lusty appetites, Lillian evidently went for food, as well as men, in a big way. She is said to have weighed some 200 pounds.

Dance revolutionary Isadora Duncan won world acclaim for her looks as well as her genius. She was hailed as a goddess of beauty by the great sculptor Rodin and countless other enthusiasts. Yet photographs show that Isadora in her prime was quite plump. The great modern choreographer George Balanchine once called her "a fat lady rolling around the stage."

THE SHIFT TOWARD THIN

It's hard to pinpoint the time exactly, but the American attitude toward feminine beauty probably began to shift in the early 1920s.

The country was enjoying exceptional prosperity. Technology was making giant strides, clearing a path for rapid and sometimes drastic social changes. Old values and sexual role models were coming into question. The woman's suffrage movement was stirring turmoil in politics.

Giddy with new freedom, women began to jettison some of the trappings of the traditional female. They bobbed their hair and shortened their skirts. Consciously or not, they began to take on a certain resemblance to the males whose dominance they challenged. They bound their breasts to achieve a fashionable flatness. They wore chemise-style dresses that obscured their waists and camouflaged their hips.

In short, the skinny Venus had arrived. And she remains today, planted on her pedestal with willowy firmness.

WHERE FAT IS STILL FINE

Unquestionably, slenderness is today's mainstream beauty standard in America, Western Europe, and most other high-technology cultures. But this is not usually the case in more primitive societies.

Scientists looking into the matter surveyed twenty-five tribal cultures. Of these, twenty had a definite preference for plump women, while only five favored thin ones. The tribes admiring roundness cut broadly across ethnic and geographical lines, ranging from some American Indians to the Bushmen of Africa.

Accounting for tastes is always tricky. But it may be that less developed cultures look for their women to be functional as well as ornamental. When females are expected to carry gear on long journeys or help in sowing and harvesting, being sturdy may well be an asset. Or it may be that fat women are rare, and therefore valuable, in areas where it's not so easy to be well nourished.

Then again, the persistent taste for fat women may have something to do with the stasis and stability of slow-to-change tribal cultures. Closer to nature and to their own roots than we are, these people may simply be more at home with the natural roundness of the female form. Like our own distant ancestors, they may value the life-giving and nurturing properties that a ripely feminine figure suggests.

WHY THINGS CHANGED: THE ECONOMICS OF BEAUTY

Given the popularity of fat historically and geographically, why do we modern Americans prize thinness so much? And if our standard of beauty is so unusual, what does this say about our culture in general?

Theories about these questions are many, and often subtle, and I'll discuss some of them at length in Chapter 10. But we can unearth some basic answers now by going back to our beginnings and tracing the way certain tastes developed.

It's obvious from the outset that notions of beauty are closely linked with laws of economics. What people find valuable, they also tend to find beautiful. A thing is valuable if it contributes to survival and prosperity. If the thing is hard to get, it becomes more valuable still.

Fat was beautiful originally for two reasons. First, it had immense survival value. Second, it was exclusive. When fat was scarce, being fat was a rarity, a sign of special status.

Fat and Survival

It took a million years or so for man to evolve from a stooped little rock-chunker to a big-brained and upright creature that we can recognize today as an ancient cousin. He started off in Africa, where the weather was warm and the living was more or less easy. But in time he expanded his turf northward into Europe and Asia.

While he was migrating, the world's weather took a nasty turn for the worse. Born in a time of tropical lushness, man came of age in a time of snow and ice. Over much of his terrain, it got very cold indeed. Faced with the climate's challenge, man had to adapt or die. One of the ways he adapted was by getting bigger and fatter.

Scientists know that animals in cold climates tend to be bigger than those in warm climates. This is true of people, just as it is of whales and polar bears. Our Ice Age ancestors helped preserve themselves by learning to store fat. It helped them keep warm, and it gave them a portable food supply when vegetation was absent and game was scarce.

The thin tended to die out, while the better-protected fat people tended to survive and reproduce. Over the centuries, then, a genetic preference for fat was built into mankind's makeup. And an aesthetic preference went with it. In proving valuable, fat also proved beautiful.

Even though tastes have changed, the hereditary bias for fat lives on today, tormenting the modern descendants of those Ice Age survivors. As well it might. It was only 12,000 years ago that the glacial period finally waned in northern Europe, a mere blink of an eye as evolutionary time is measured.

Fat, the Portable Pantry

We humans have probably always been omnivorous creatures. That means we eat almost anything.

When mankind was first starting his evolutionary climb, he probably enjoyed a fairly plentiful and varied warm-weather diet. He could eat fruit off the trees and berries off the bushes. He ate meat as well, as long as it was easy to get. Unfortunately, this was seldom the case. Man was a rather puny creature, not up to hunting in competition with bigger, stronger, and faster animals.

But if he was smaller and slower, man was also smarter. When hard times came and plant life got scarce, he developed tools and strategies that made him a successful hunter. Animal protein became his chief cuisine.

He may have had to go days, even weeks, between kills. But his ability to store fat helped see him through the lean times. By gorging himself when hunting was good, he was able to lay in enough fuel to keep him going until the next kill.

Again, fat ensured survival. And again, nature took note and programmed the fat-storing tendency into man's genes.

Fat, Sex, and Female Status

The division of labor in the Old Stone Age was necessarily simple. There was no agriculture. Men hunted. Women bore children and kept things in order around the house — or, more accurately, around the cave.

Women could eat what little they could glean from the scanty vegetation. But in the main, men controlled the food supply. What meat they didn't eat on the hunt, they brought home for distribution to the women and children.

It's likely that the largest share of the leftovers went to the women the hunters found most attractive. Since it was these women who therefore had the best chance to get fat, fatness probably became a sign of sexiness and favored status. The association was self-perpetuating: sexy women got fat, and fat women were considered sexy. It's no wonder, then, that the prodigiously pudgy Venus of Willendorf was the sex symbol of her age.

It's also likely that fatness was deemed valuable and beautiful because it was associated with fertility. The association is based on biological fact, which even the primitive caveman could observe. It takes a certain amount of body fat for a woman to conceive, bear, and nourish a child. The fatter women of the Stone Age probably had fewer miscarriages and stillbirths, and produced more and healthier babies, than their thinner sisters.

This was a crucial ability. It was an age when the rigors of life allowed few women to survive to the age of thirty. The time for breeding was short, so children were at a premium. Fertile females were cherished, and the fatter they were, the better.

Best of all were the fat women who carried much of their weight in their breasts. Because of their role in feeding the young, breasts were probably also a part of the fertility fetish that inspired worship in our prehistoric forebears.

Beauty and Scarcity

So much for the caveman and his mate. But why did the taste for fatness persist so long, surviving the Stone Age by thousands of years?

Because the same basic economic law of supply and demand was still at work. What's scarce is valuable. The shorter the supply, the more desirable the commodity. This is true of gold, diamonds, oil, and — depending on conditions — fatness or leanness.

And the fact is that food, and fatness, remained relative rarities for a very long time.

The rigors of the Stone Age were extreme, of course, and they eased somewhat as tool-making became more sophisticated and agriculture arose. Nomadic wanderings gave way to settlements, towns, and cities. Trade and commerce flowered.

But for the great mass of humanity, progress was only marginal. Even in the richest of ancient civilizations, comfort and plenty were enjoyed only by a few. The vast majority of people remained poor, surviving at little better than sustenance level. Wars, plagues, and famines were monotonous recurrences that disrupted whole populations and economies.

In short, mankind enjoyed very few plush times and many centuries of scarcity.

Only with the coming of the Industrial Revolution some 130 years ago did prosperity become even faintly democratic, and then only in advanced nations. Up until then, most people worked very hard for very little, and getting fat was a luxury few could afford.

Under such conditions, fatness remained a sign of success, status, and favor, just as it was for the curvy cave lady. Fat was associated with food, survival, sexiness, and other desirable things, so fat itself was desirable. Fat was beautiful.

Beauty and Plenty

When times are hard, fat is beautiful, and times have usually been hard.

But what happens when times are easy?

The answer is obvious. Fat loses both its survival value and its exclusivity. Fat becomes ugly. Thin becomes beautiful.

We Americans bear witness to this turnabout. We're among the richest people in the world, among the fattest, and certainly among those most obsessed with losing weight. We're rivaled in poundage only by our similarly rich European cousins, who also despise fat and want to be thin.

For us, food is abundant and relatively cheap. Few people miss meals, except by choice, and fewer still need ever fear starvation. Undernourishment was yesterday's health threat. Overnourishment is today's. Far from helping us survive, the fat resulting from too much food, obtained with too little physical labor, poses a major danger to modern man (see Chapter 4).

In addition to being no longer helpful, fatness is no longer rare. Almost anybody can get fat in our bountiful society, and many people do. There's nothing exclusive about being fat in America, where between 25 and 35 percent of the adult population is overweight to some degree.

As a result, fatness has become common, in every sense of the word. No longer a symbol of elegance, being fat is now deemed dowdy, dumpy, disgusting, slovenly, and lower-class. To many, it indicates weak will and gluttonous self-indulgence. In the prevailing view today, fat *is* ugly.

FAT AND SELF-IMAGE TODAY

It may be a sign of just how rich we are that slimness in America today is more than just a matter of taste. It has become an ethic, an obsession, and a cult. There's no other way to explain why weight control in this country is such big business, or why, at any given moment, at least 20 million Americans are on reducing diets.

The obsession sometimes translates into ego-battering ridicule and discrimination directed against overweight people.

If you're overweight yourself, the societal bias can be hard to take. But don't let it add the extra burden of guilt to your extra pounds. Being overweight doesn't say anything about your basic worth as a person. It doesn't necessarily mean that you're self-indulgent or gluttonous or un-controlled — or even that you're "ugly." All it says for sure about you as a social being is that you're swimming against the current tide of aesthetic preference.

It's true that anybody who eats little enough and stays active enough will lose weight. If one keeps up such a regimen forever, one will stay thin forever. But it's also true that some people are genetically pro-grammed to store fat easily, and they have to fight very hard to stay thin. Moreover, women generally have a tougher time of it than men. You shouldn't use your genes or your gender to minimize the importance of excess weight. But you're justified in taking them into account if you're looking for a place to lay the blame.

FAT IN PERSPECTIVE

Your first step in solving a weight problem is to see it for what it primarily is — a medical consideration, not a cosmetic one. You should shed excess pounds mainly because they can hurt your health, not because modern taste decrees that they're unattractive.

I don't mean to minimize the toll that fat can take on your psyche in a world that treasures slimness. But aesthetics should be a secondary consideration. Don't make yourself miserable dwelling on your failure to conform to some current, and possibly temporary, norm of what's "beautiful."

Remember: despite the current trend, there's nothing innately ugly about fat — as the popularity of fat women throughout history proves.

You may find scant consolation in the fact that larger women were much admired in the past, or that they still are in some cultures other than our own. After all, you live here and now — not in a prehistoric cave or a modern igloo. Prevailing taste is the one you must contend with.

Still, a little perspective should help the next time you're inclined to compare yourself unfavorably to some fashion model whose hipbones are holding up her high-style skirt. In almost any other age, you would have been the one whose body was considered beautiful and sexy. People would have found more of famine than of femininity in the skinny Venus you envy today.

3.

FAT AS A FRIEND

If it weren't for body fat, camels couldn't cross the desert. Seals couldn't reproduce. Birds couldn't migrate. Bears couldn't survive a cold winter.

As for you and me, we'd totter in listless desperation from water tap to water tap, too weak to do much else. We probably wouldn't survive long — not as individuals and not as a species. Along with outsized brains and opposable thumbs, our ability to store body fat has been a major asset in bringing us so far in the evolutionary scheme of things.

Today, the protective advantages of fat may seem outdated — about as useful as the muscles we still have for wagging a long-vanished tail.

But you never know. This era is no more than the tick of a second on the clock that measures aeons. Want, not plenty, has been the customary lot of most of mankind over the centuries. The time may come again when fat will prove its worth.

THE VALUE OF FAT

As you may already realize from what I've said so far, body fat is vital for human survival. For us and for virtually all other creatures that move, it's a portable storehouse for both water and energy. In addition, fat provides insulation against the cold and a reserve for females to draw on in bearing and feeding their young. In the worst of crises, stored fat can help protect your brain.

Water

The most famous portable water tank around belongs to the camel. This ungainly creature can plod the burning desert sands for a week or longer without a drink of water because it carries its own water supply, in the form of a hump. The hump is no more than a large lump of fat that undergoes chemical breakdown, or metabolism, as the camel proceeds on its waterless trek.

To understand how the camel manages this considerable feat, you need to know a little more about metabolism.

Almost every one of the trillions of cells in your body (and the camel's) is a tiny reactor. This reactor continually takes in complex chemical substances and breaks them down into increasingly simpler substances.

In camels and in us, one of the substances produced from this step-by-step breakdown of the original substances into simpler ones is water. The water yield of fat is high — every gram of fat that is subjected to the step-down process of metabolism produces 1.2 milliliters of water. This means that the camel's hump can supply the camel with upwards of 80 liters or 160 pounds of water between drinks.

By journey's end, the hump has flattened out to become a loose flap of skin hanging on the camel's back. But with some food and a long drink of water, the hump fills and rises, and the animal is ready for the next dry spell.

Humans can use either stored sugar or stored fat as a source of water, but fat is better. It yields twice as much water per gram as stored sugar. If it weren't for the ability to metabolize stored fat for water, humans couldn't exist for very long away from a water source. You'd have to drink almost continuously to supply your body's constant need for this most essential commodity.

Energy

Just as you can use sugar or fat to produce water, you can use either one to provide energy when no food is available. Again, fat is by far the better source.

In the same way it produces water, the chemical activity of metabolism also produces energy. Oxygen helps fuel the breakdown process, just as it feeds a fire, so we say that the cells "burn" substances to create energy. Like fire, which produces energy in the form of heat and light, chemical breakdown or "burning" in the cells produces energy to fuel movement and all other life processes.

SUGAR

Sugar, which comes from many of the foods you eat, is one form of raw material for the cellular reactors to work on. As sugar is gradually broken down into simpler and simpler substances, energy is released in the process. If the sugar is completely processed, this continues until the simplest by-products of all are reached — carbon dioxide and water.

These two substances are released back into your bloodstream for eventual elimination. You breathe off carbon dioxide and water vapor when you exhale. More excess water circulates to your kidneys for elimination in your urine.

Your body prefers using sugar to using fat as an energy source for two reasons.

First, sugar is easier to process. It breaks down into simple components easily and completely, leaving no leftovers. Fat, as you will see, leaves some debris behind when it burns. You might compare sugar to the gasoline that's better suited to your car engine than crude oil. The engine can burn up all the gasoline but the crude oil would leave messy, unburned leftovers.

The second advantage of sugar is that it burns with a minimum of oxygen. Fat requires a lot more. This is why your body uses sugar almost exclusively during heavy exercise. In a hard workout, you use up so much oxygen, so fast, that the cells lack the oxygen they need to burn fat efficiently.

Despite its advantages, there's a major problem with sugar as an energy source: you can't store very much of it.

Sugar is stored in your muscles, your liver, and your bloodstream. At any given time, the average person has about 10 grams of sugar in his bloodstream. This is only about 40 calories' worth of energy. The liver stores another 50 grams, or 200 calories, and the muscles about 125 grams, or 500 calories.

The total storage capacity, then, comes to a meager 750 calories — not nearly enough to satisfy your energy needs for a single day.

FAT

When sugar runs short, or when you're resting, your body burns mostly fat for energy. The great virtue of fat is that it's very easy to store and to carry in large amounts. You're built to warehouse fat, not sugar.

Your body has vast fat depots, including your liver and all the areas under your skin and around your internal organs. The average person has from 12 to 30 pounds of body fat, which translates into 42,000 to 105,000 calories.

If you relied only on your stored sugar to provide life-sustaining energy in the absence of food, you would die in one day. But with your fat reserves to tap, you could survive without food for about sixty days.

As you've seen, your body ordinarily burns mostly sugar during periods of demanding physical activity. But when you're at rest, and your oxygen supply is high, your body burns fat — wisely drawing on the more plentiful energy source. (Not that you can get thin lying in bed. As you'll learn in detail in Chapter 11, what matters in weight loss is how many calories you use up, not their source.)

Again, you can think of your internal energy needs in terms of energy in the environment. We prefer to burn oil instead of coal because oil is generally cleaner and more efficient. But we still try to burn coal whenever possible because oil is in short supply while coal is abundant. Similarly, our bodies may prefer using sugar as a fuel. But it's efficient in the long run to use as much fat as possible, simply because there's so much more of it.

I'll have more to say about fat metabolism later in explaining how fat stores can help preserve your brain.

FAT'S ENERGY EFFICIENCY

Plentiful, portable body fat is good news for the male Alaskan fur seal, whose best friend is his blubber. This animal lives ten months of the year in the frigid sea, gobbling everything he can lay a flipper on. He's laying in a lavish store of fat. He needs it when he goes ashore.

In the summer, the seals go on land for two months. There the seal pups are born, and the new mating season begins. The female seals become fertile right after giving birth.

The mature seal bull has a harem of cows, usually around a hundred. When he isn't laboring to inseminate them all, he's busy fending off would-be poachers from the contingent of young bachelor seals. With all this ferocious fighting and procreating, the bull seal neither eats nor sleeps for two solid months. By the time he once again waddles gratefully seaward, he's about 200 pounds lighter. Had he not been able to store that excess poundage, his genes would have gone uncontributed. And he would have had a very dull summer.

Fat as they get, seals never come close to the body-fat percentages of migratory birds. Preparing for their winter treks to warmer climates, these birds stuff themselves. During the two weeks before takeoff their body fat may increase to ten times its normal proportion. They have special storage depots in their bellies and backs to hold the extra fuel, which powers them on flights that can cover thousands of miles.

Of course, humans need never carry around such large reserves. You certainly don't need them in America, where missed meals are usually a matter of choice, not necessity. But your body is unaware of prevailing conditions. It continues to provide you with a fat layer to see you through whatever hard times might come. It gives you the potential to "feed on yourself" to sustain life for as long as several weeks without food.

Even though you'll never face a famine, your fat stores let you get through the day with enough energy to last from meal to meal, and through the night with no food at all. And, unless you're grossly over-weight, your fat is easy to carry and obligingly plastic. It molds easily around your bones and organs, and it fits into whatever odd-shaped space you choose to put it.

Insulation

Just as it's a sort of portable water bucket and fuel tank, your stored fat is also a movable blanket. It stands between the elements and your vital and vulnerable internal organs, which must be kept warm.

In addition to providing cover against the cold, the fat also manufactures heat. Heat is another form of the energy produced by the metabolizing of fat.

It is this function that causes bears to put on mounds of fat in the fall to draw on during a winter of hibernation or extreme inactivity. The fat both nourishes and warms them in a time of scarcity and cold.

Like its other functions, this warming role of fat may be passé in this era of year-round climate control. But your genes know nothing of such newfangled gadgets as central heat and air conditioning. They heed the logic of thousands of years of evolution aimed at protecting the odd, hairless mammals that we are against an environment that could kill us. A dozen generations of indoor heat can hardly erase a genetic memory of cold stretching all the way back to the last Ice Age.

Reproduction

Spurred on by her hormones, a pregnant woman usually gains weight whether she wants to or not — weight well in excess of the weight of the fetus she's carrying.

And well she should. The extra energy the fat provides is necessary to help her meet the increased demands made on her own body, as well as the needs of the infant.

Since the unborn baby has hardly any fat of its own until shortly before birth, it depends almost entirely on its mother for nourishment and heat. The mother has to pump more blood, process more food, and, in general, do everything needed to accommodate two bodies instead of one.

After the baby is born, the mother still needs the extra fat she has accumulated. A hormone called *prolactin* helps mobilize it to her breasts, where it's used in the production of milk.

A mother who doesn't store enough fat in the course of her pregnancy is at risk of having an underweight baby. An infant with a low birthweight is much more likely to suffer brain damage, retardation, infection, and a host of diseases that afflict newborns.

This fact has made most obstetricians ease up on the maternal weight-gain restrictions that were fashionable only a few years ago. The doctors might have learned the lesson sooner had they heeded nature's own attitude toward excessive thinness: when a woman's body-fat percentage falls too low, she becomes unable to get pregnant. (See Chapter 9 for more on fat and reproduction.)

Brain Preservation

This last item is mostly of academic interest, since none of us is ever likely to starve. But it illustrates how wonderfully your body is equipped, even in the worst of times, to protect its most precious single asset, the brain.

At any time, your brain gets royally preferential treatment. It receives a hugely disproportionate share of blood and oxygen relative to its size, even if other organs have to suffer to supply it. Fat nourishes your other tissues much of the time. But the brain dines almost exclusively on sugar, which, you'll remember, is in much shorter supply.

However, if prolonged malnourishment limits the amount of available sugar, the brain can still survive for a time on energy supplied by *ketones*. Ketones are the fat-metabolism "leftovers" that I mentioned earlier.

KETONES

Ketones are fragments of incompletely burned fat. This is how they are produced:

When your body runs low on sugar, it has to meet its energy needs by calling up fat from cells in your fat storage depots. The fat enters your bloodstream and goes to other cells, which burn it for energy.

The fat components that are burned are called *fatty acids*. There are scores of different fatty acids, but all can end up as carbon dioxide and water — if they're broken down completely.

Large amounts of the fatty acids traveling in your bloodstream are picked up by your liver. The liver uses them for energy, or stores them as potential energy for the future. But the liver can't break down the fatty acids completely. There are leftovers — the ketones.

The liver releases ketones back into the bloodstream. They travel to the muscles, the kidneys, and the brain, which are the only tissues that can finish breaking them down into carbon dioxide and water.

But complete ketone breakdown can only go so fast. If your body is burning fat almost exclusively over a period of time, the liver puts out more ketones than the muscles, kidneys, and brain can handle. The ketones then build up in the bloodstream.

Ketones can build up if you're short on sugar because you haven't eaten in several hours, or because you're on a low-carbohydrate diet. The same thing happens if you have a disease such as diabetes that prevents your using sugar. If the ketone buildup goes on long enough— as it would if you were starving — the ketones can reach toxic levels and make you very sick.

But at the same time, the ketones do a vital service in this desperate state. They nourish your brain. Brain cells can break down ketones for energy, so your brain will accept them as food when there's not enough sugar to supply it. By providing ketones, your body contrives to keep your brain going until the last possible minute, even if you're starving to death. In starvation, people die of heart failure, never of brain death.

THANK HEAVEN FOR FAT

Being thin may be the most cherished goal of your life, and you may think you hate everything about fat. But don't be too quick to knock it.

Our current abundance of food means that for now, fat appears to have outlived its usefulness in many ways. But fat isn't intrinsically bad, any more than it's intrinsically ugly. It's bad only when you have so much of it that your health is endangered.

Otherwise, fat deserves a little gratitude. Water, energy, warmth, fertility, and the capacity for thought are the gifts of life itself. And fat can provide all of them. That's why we have it in the first place.

4.

FAT AS AN ENEMY

To the extent that it's natural and necessary, body fat is a good thing. But like most good things, having too much of it can cause problems. In the case of too much fat, the problems can be severe.

Leaving aside for now the damage that extra pounds inflict on your ego, consider the more important matter of what they do to your body.

Being underweight or overweight is potentially unhealthy, of course, but being overweight is worse. *Underweight is an indication of harmful conditions. Overweight is a harmful condition in itself.*

HEALTH PROBLEMS AND FAT

Being overweight is associated with "degenerative" diseases, or those that break down body tissue. Your body simply isn't equipped to handle an overload of flesh for any length of time, and there are many ways it can break down under the strain.

It's true that being fat can't always be pinpointed as the direct cause of degenerative illnesses. But it's safe to say that certain conditions associated with fat are also associated with these diseases. For instance, being fat may not in itself cause heart attacks. But high levels of certain blood fats do contribute to heart attacks, and fat people often have high blood-fat levels.

Your Heart

Many of the early deaths that happen to fat people result from cardiovascular disease. Researchers estimate that at least one fourth of all problems involving the heart and blood vessels are connected with being fat. The main reason for this, as I just noted, is that people with excess fat on their bodies often have excess fat in their blood as well.

CHOLESTEROL AND PLAQUE

Fat people take in more calories than they need, and the extra calories are all converted by the liver to fat. The fat can take several forms, depending on how it is to be used by the body later. For instance, it can become triglycerides, the blood fat that you burn for energy or store for later use.

Health Disorders Associated with Obesity

HEART
Heart attacks
Heart pain
Congestive heart failure

BLOOD VESSELS
High blood pressure
Strokes
Varicose veins
Hemorrhoids
Clots

SKIN
Stretch marks
Rash under the arms and
in the groin from abrasion

LIVER
Gallstones
Fatty livers

KIDNEY
Kidney failure

BONES AND JOINTS
Arthritis

SEXUAL FUNCTION AND REPRODUCTION
Increased risk of diabetes and
high blood pressure during pregnancy
Reduced fertility
Irregular menstruation

CANCER
Cancer of the uterus
Cancer of the breast
Cancer of the prostate
Cancer of the colon

DISEASES
Diabetes
Gout

MISCELLANEOUS
Accident proneness
Increased surgical risks
Decreased immunity to disease

The liver can also convert excess calories to a kind of blood fat called *cholesterol*. There are two types of cholesterol, one beneficial and one destructive. The beneficial kind is called *high-density lipoprotein*, or HDL. The bad kind is called *low-density lipoprotein*, or LDL.

HDL helps maintain your arteries, the vessels that carry blood from the heart to the rest of the body. This cholesterol helps keep the arteries free of material that can narrow them and rob them of their elasticity.

LDL — the one you hear about in connection with heart attacks — is exactly the opposite. It can become embedded in the artery walls, hardening there to form a material called *plaque*. The buildup of layers of plaque can narrow the arteries, restricting the flow of blood through them.

HIGH BLOOD PRESSURE

Narrow arteries increase the resistance the heart must work against as it pumps blood through the body. The greater the resistance, the higher the blood pressure.

You can picture this clearly if you compare an artery to a garden hose. If you cover half the mouth of the hose with your hand, water comes out of the remaining half with much greater force. Similarly, blood trying to make its way through arteries partially blocked by plaque is traveling at high pressure.

Not only does plaquing create high blood pressure; high blood pressure can lead in turn to more plaquing. The increased pressure wears down the inner walls of the arteries, creating worn spots that are targets for the deposit of more plaque.

People process their food in different ways, depending on such factors as gender and heredity. Some are more susceptible than others to developing high cholesterol levels. But for many victims of obesity, extra calories end up as high cholesterol, which brings on plaquing and high blood pressure. It can hardly be a coincidence that as doctors at Northwestern University Medical School in Chicago found, high blood pressure afflicts twice as many fat people as people of normal weight.

STROKE, HEART ATTACK, AND KIDNEY FAILURE

High blood pressure and plaquing can lead to stroke, heart attack, and kidney failure.

The tissue that makes up your vital organs — including your brain, heart, and kidneys — stays alive through a constant supply of oxygen-bearing blood. Deprived of an adequate amount of blood, the tissue dies.

If the blood flow in arteries leading to your brain is diminished because of plaquing, brain tissue dies from oxygen starvation. This is what happens when someone suffers a stroke. Inadequate blood flow to the brain can also be a cause of senility in older people.

If the arteries feeding the heart itself become choked with plaque, an area of the heart tissue will be starved of its blood supply. If this happens, that area of the heart dies (this is what a heart attack is). Similarly, kidney failure can result if the kidneys don't get enough blood, which provides them with the oxygen they need to function properly.

Along with blocking arteries, plaque weakens them and makes them rigid. They can no longer expand and contract elastically with the pulsing flow of blood. As this happens, they become increasingly vulnerable to the eroding effects of high blood pressure and additional plaquing.

Eventually, a worn artery wall can give way altogether, completely disrupting the blood supply to the organ that artery feeds. Again, the result can be a crippling or lethal stroke, heart attack, or kidney shutdown.

Other Ailments

Your cardiovascular system is by no means the only part of your body endangered by excess poundage.

Obesity renders you four times more likely to contract diabetes. It makes you more subject to arthritis and more likely to develop certain liver disorders. If you're a woman, it creates problems with pregnancy and childbirth, and it increases your risk of contracting uterine cancer.

Being overweight undermines your immune system. It makes you more vulnerable to gallstones. It promotes blood clots and varicose veins.

These are among the more serious hazards you're courting if you're overweight. (For a complete list of obesity-related conditions, see page 28.)

DIABETES

Fat people are vulnerable to diabetes because of abnormalities involving the hormone insulin.

Insulin is produced by the pancreas. Its main function is to drive sugar and fat out of your bloodstream and into cells. The sugar can go into virtually any cell of your body. Most of the fat goes into specialized cells, called *fat cells*, for storage. In aggregate, these fat cells make up your body's fat storage depots.

The fatter you are, the fuller your fat cells are. When they're full, they resist taking in any more fat. So your body steps up insulin production in an uphill effort to keep your blood clear.

But even as the pancreas is pouring out more and more insulin, the fat person is becoming less and less sensitive to it. Eventually, the insulin is ineffective for herding either fat or sugar out of the blood and into cells. This insensitivity to insulin constitutes the most common form of diabetes.

Fortunately, weight loss alone can often cure this type of diabetes. Losing weight empties some of the fat cells, so the person is once again able to respond to insulin.

(For more information on insulin and how it promotes fat storage, see Chapter 6.)

ARTHRITIS
Osteoarthritis, a disease involving the breakdown of the cartilage lining the joints, is common among the overweight.

Fat people are usually inactive, and bones and cartilage require the stress of exercise to help them retain the mineral calcium that helps keep them strong. In addition, being overweight aggravates osteoarthritis by putting extra strain on the weight-bearing joints such as the hips and knees.

FATTY LIVER
A very fat person tends to accumulate an undue amount of fat in the liver. Through some unknown mechanism, this excess fat can cause scarring of the liver. The scarring can impede the liver's vital function of governing the way the body processes food. (Technically, this scarring is called *cirrhosis*.)

DISEASES OF PREGNANCY
During pregnancy, fat women are far more likely than normal-weight women to suffer from high blood pressure and diabetes. High blood pressure can lead to stunted fetal growth, and diabetes to several birth defects.

DIFFICULT DELIVERIES AND INFERTILITY

Obese mothers-to-be tend to have more difficulty doing the hard work of labor and delivery because they are less fit. And recent research connects obesity with several menstrual-cycle disorders, including decreased ovulation, that can result in infertility.

CANCER IN WOMEN

Obese women are more likely to develop cancer of the uterus and breast. Both of these tissues grow when stimulated by the female hormone estrogen. Another female hormone, called progesterone, limits this response to estrogen.

Obese women often do not release an egg each month, and the release of an egg is necessary for the production of progesterone. If no egg is released, no progesterone is made.

It is the lack of progesterone that increases a woman's chance of developing cancer of the uterus and, possibly, also of the breast. If there is no progesterone to limit the estrogen-stimulation of the breast and uterus, these tissues may grow uncontrollably — and uncontrolled cell growth is cancer.

If you are obese and menstruate every twenty-six to thirty days, chances are that you are not more likely to develop cancer of the uterus or breast. But if you are obese and menstruate at irregular intervals, you should check with your doctor. He or she can tell whether you are making enough estrogen to increase your chances of getting cancer of the uterus. This can be determined by performing a simple blood test or by examining the mucus coming from your cervix, the mouth of the uterus. Estrogen causes the cervix to produce large amounts of clear, watery mucus.

DECREASED IMMUNITY

Your immune system is a complex bodily network that helps protect you against invading organisms — viruses, bacteria, and even carcinogens. Everyone's immune system becomes less effective with age, but it appears that obesity hastens the deterioration. Researchers are not yet sure why this is so, but the fact itself is well established.

GALLSTONES

As you know, obese people are likely to have high blood levels of cholesterol. Some of this cholesterol is picked up by the liver and routed down to the gallbladder for storage as a component of bile. The gall-bladder periodically squeezes the bile into the intestines, where it speeds the absorption of certain vitamins and helps clear away excess fat you take in from fatty food.

Too much cholesterol in the blood can wind up as excess cholesterol in the bile. In this case, the cholesterol can become so concentrated in the liquid bile that part of it solidifies and forms stones.

The stones rub against the inner lining of the gallbladder, and may even block the passage of bile from the gallbladder to the intestines. The result is a painful, swollen gallbladder, which must sometimes be re-moved surgically.

The only good news here is that the gallbladder is not a vital organ; you can get along without it.

BLOOD CLOTS

Blood clots are always dangerous, and they can be life-threatening if they choke off the blood supply in an artery feeding a vital organ.

Doctors aren't sure why fat people are more likely to get blood clots. The probable reason is that overweight people usually get little or no regular exercise.

Exercise stimulates production of a protein that discourages clotting. As nonexercisers, obese people don't benefit from this anticlotting mechanism.

VARICOSE VEINS

Your arteries carry blood away from the heart; your veins carry blood back to it. The veins are aided in this job by tiny valves that line their inner walls. The valves open and close, forming a one-way route to keep blood moving in the right direction. If a vein's valves don't work properly, blood can pool in the vein and stretch it. A vein widened in this way is called a *varicose* vein.

Veins are located in the fat layer between the muscles and the skin. Ordinarily, the tautness of the skin on one side and of the muscles on the other exerts pressure to help keep the veins constricted and the valves in good working order.

But spongy fat tissue offers much less resistance than skin or muscle. If your fat layer is very thick, the veins inside it are more likely to expand. As a vein widens, the valves inside it are no longer large enough to close completely as they move the blood along. Blood can leak backward, stretching the vein even more.

This circulatory problem is common among overweight people.

ACCIDENTS AND POSTOPERATIVE PROBLEMS

Along with being easy prey to many illnesses, fat people are more susceptible to complications after surgery. They come down with more postoperative infections, and it takes longer for their surgical wounds to heal.

Finally, studies show that excess fat causes people to be clumsier and slower in their reaction times than thinner people. The obese suffer a disproportionate share of accidents, including auto mishaps.

LIFE SPANS

Being fat can shorten your life as well as impair your health. The fatter you are, the more likely you are to reduce your life span. This is the conclusion of virtually all studies ever done of the effects of obesity on longevity. For example, statistics compiled by the Metropolitan Life Insurance Company show that a man of forty-five carrying 25 pounds of excess fat cuts his life expectancy by 25 percent.

As you can see, then, being fat is serious business from a medical point of view. There's a lot more at stake than how you look in your bikini, or how dashing a figure you cut on the tennis court.

If you're still battling to take weight off, hang in there.

If you're at your proper weight, be thankful and stay there.

And if you're not sure what "proper weight" means for you, read on. You're about to find out.

5.

ARE YOU TOO FAT?

You look in a full-length mirror, and you hate what you see.

You step on the scales. The dial spins and slows, ominous as a roulette wheel about to give you the bad news. The numbers come up. You're horrified. The conclusion is inescapable.

"I'm fat," you moan.

You may very well be right. But so far, you haven't done anything to prove it. Scales won't tell you if you're fat. Neither will your eyes. Neither will height-weight charts.

Amazingly, you may not even be able to get doctors to agree on whether you're too fat. Obesity is a major medical problem in America. Tons of research have been done on it. Yet doctors often write hundreds of pages about it without ever telling you exactly what it is.

DEFINITIONS—NOT AS EASY AS YOU THINK

The questions seem so simple: What is an "ideal" weight? How much can you deviate from the ideal before you're "fat"? What does "fat" mean?

The questions are simple; the answers aren't.

Researchers have tried to establish weight "norms" in a number of ways. They've experimented with nutrition plans, with exercise programs, with humans, with animals. They've surveyed large populations to see how weight relates to health and long life.

But after all this, "norms" still don't mean much to any one weight-watcher. They're too arbitrary. There will always be quite a few individuals who don't have a weight problem, but who still don't fit the charts and graphs.

Just Looking

Chances are that if you think you look fat, you are fat. A bulge over the beltline is probably telling you something. But not always. You may see yourself as a good ten pounds over your best bathing suit weight and still be well within the limits set by science as ideal. On the other hand, you may look quite thin and still carry too much fat over tiny bones and muscles.

So much for the eye of the beholder.

Scales and Charts

Like the naked eye, weight scales and height-weight charts are only signposts. All they can do is help *indicate* that you're too fat. They can't tell you for sure.

The fault with both scales and charts is that they measure the wrong thing. They measure weight, not fat. And weight is not the right criterion for judging obesity.

Bones and muscles weigh much more than fat. If you're large-boned and muscular, you'll exceed most "ideal" weights laid out by insurance companies and diet-book authors. Even so, you'll have very little body fat. It's perfectly possible for a sleek ballerina to weigh more than a sedentary woman who looks, and is, too fat.

The legendary Russian weight lifter Vasily Alexeev is a little over six feet tall and weighs around 330 pounds. He looks enormously fat. His weight testifies that he's fat. Yet his body fat accounts for less than 12 percent of that weight. The rest is bone and mammoth muscle. Vasily Alexeev is not too fat.

VARIATIONS IN THE CHARTS

You veteran dieters are probably well acquainted with the height-weight tables that purport to give you your ideal weight based on your height and sex. Some of the charts factor in age and body build as well.

You've probably noticed that these tables don't always agree with one another. Recommended weights may vary by several pounds. One reason is that each chart's author may incorporate anything from clinical experience to personal taste in arriving at a particular "ideal." The reader seldom has any way of knowing, or judging, what factors applied.

In any case, all the tables are artificial. They may help give you some idea of how you stack up against some fictional norm, but all are generalizations that make little allowance for individual body variations.

And again, all deal with weight, not fat. So even the best of the charts, most carefully arrived at, is no more than a guide.

THE BUILD AND BLOOD PRESSURE STUDIES

The best of the guides are probably those based on two massive studies done by the Society of Actuaries between the years of 1935 and 1972. They were called the Build and Blood Pressure Studies (BBPS), and they were used by the Metropolitan Life Insurance Company as an aid in setting insurance rates.

The purpose of the studies was to determine what body weights were most conducive to good health and long life.

BBPS researchers followed millions of people over a period of years to arrive at their findings. Those findings were, of course, that higher weights were associated with impaired health and shortened life spans.

The insurance company used the findings to set up height-weight tables of the sort you see in diet books today.

The BBPS tables are the best you're likely to find because the research that went into them was sweeping and solid. But they, too, are merely a guide. They deal with weight, not fat.

THE FRAMINGHAM STUDY

Despite their flaws, the BBPS tables were widely accepted by many scientists for research purposes until just recently.

In 1980, the *Journal of the American Medical Association* published the Framingham Study. This survey, which had been commissioned by the National Institutes of Health, followed 5,209 residents of Framingham, Massachusetts, over a period of some thirty years. Its findings differed in some respects from those of the venerated BBPS.

Most significantly, the Framingham Study, which used longevity as its standard, came up with ideal weights that were 7 percent to 10 percent *higher* than those established by the BBPS.

For instance, the healthiest weight for a 5'9" man according to the BBPS was 146 pounds. The Framingham Study, however, determined that a 5'9" man who weighed 170 pounds lived longer than men of that height who weighed more, or less, than 170 pounds. Similarly, the BBPS said a 5'6" woman should weigh 130 pounds. But the Framingham Study's research concluded that to live longer, a 5'6" woman should

THE BBPS GUIDE TO WEIGHT BY HEIGHT AND AGE

The figures represent weights in ordinary indoor clothing and shoes, and heights with shoes.

MEN

HEIGHT	20–24	25–29	30–39	40–49	50–59	60–69
5'2"	130	134	138	140	141	140
5'3"	136	140	143	144	145	144
5'4"	139	143	147	149	150	149
5'5"	143	147	151	154	155	153
5'6"	148	152	156	158	159	158
5'7"	153	156	160	163	164	163
5'8"	157	161	165	167	168	167
5'9"	163	166	170	172	173	172
5'10"	167	171	174	176	177	176
5'11"	171	175	179	181	182	181
6'0"	176	181	184	186	187	186
6'1"	182	186	190	192	193	191
6'2"	187	191	195	197	198	196
6'3"	193	197	201	203	204	200
6'4"	198	202	206	208	209	207

WOMEN

HEIGHT	20–24	25–29	30–39	40–49	50–59	60–69
4'10"	105	110	113	118	121	123
4'11"	110	112	115	121	125	127
5'0"	112	114	118	123	127	130
5'1"	116	119	121	127	131	133
5'2"	120	121	124	129	133	136
5'3"	124	125	128	133	137	140
5'4"	127	128	131	136	141	143
5'5"	130	132	134	139	144	147
5'6"	133	134	137	143	147	150
5'7"	137	138	141	147	152	155
5'8"	141	142	145	150	156	158
5'9"	146	148	150	155	159	161
5'10"	149	150	153	158	162	163
5'11"	155	156	159	162	166	167
6'0"	157	159	164	168	171	172

1979 Build and Blood Pressure Study, published by the Society of Actuaries and the Association of Life Insurance Medical Directors of America. Reprinted with permission of the publisher.

weigh 147 pounds. (At the time this book goes to press, the tables showing the Framingham conclusions have not yet been made public.)

While scientists were puzzling over these findings, weight-watchers were rejoicing. They weren't as fat as they thought they were!

Alas, the rejoicing was at best premature, and at worst unfounded:

- Framingham was only one study. Its findings have not been substantiated by other studies, so they are by no means conclusive.
- Researchers aren't yet sure what the Framingham data mean. We don't know why the ideal weights turned out to be higher, or whether what seemed healthy in Framingham will prove to be healthier for everybody.
- The study gave higher guidelines for healthy weight, but it by no means endorsed overweight. On the contrary, it followed all other research in finding that excess weight threatened health and shortened life.
- For purposes of the individual, the study's findings are mostly academic. Once again, we have a study dealing with weight, not fat. It provides some interesting fodder for research. But it says very little to you personally about how much fat is too much fat.

If you're one of those people who celebrated Framingham's upward revision in weights, don't feel deflated now. Maybe the new charts are no cause for optimism, but then, the old ones were no cause for pessimism. Neither has any absolute meaning for you.

You'll do well to forget them both, along with every other table, chart, and graph. Instead of measuring yourself against some abstract statistic, set about finding the right weight for you and you alone.

THE REAL NORM

In this book, I throw around a lot of terms: "fat," "overweight," "obese," and "skinny," "slender," "slim," and "thin."

The last four are easy. For our purposes, being skinny, slender, slim, or thin just means not being fat. The terms mean being at, or acceptably below, an ideal percentage of body fat.

Technically, "overweight" is a misleading word. "Overfat" would be better for pinpointing the real issue. Still, "overweight" is a familiar term, and I mean it to be interchangeable with "fat" and "obese."

The sanest definition for all these terms is this: *You're fat, overweight, or obese if you have an excess of body fat sufficient to impair your health or shorten your life.*

Okay. But how much excess is sufficient to hurt you?

Figuring the Percentages

The first thing you have to do is forget about your weight as a true measure of obesity. Focus instead on how much of that weight is made up of fat.

Here's the ideal you're aiming for: *For healthy people who are not regular exercisers, the ideal body-fat percentages are 25 percent for a woman, 15 percent for a man.*

People who get regular, strenuous exercise could subtract at least 5 percentage points from those figures to arrive at their ideals — about 20 percent for women, 10 percent for men. You'll learn the exact parameters for vigorous exercise in Chapter 15. For now, consider that the 20 and 10 percent figures apply to people who have hard workouts of at least thirty minutes, at least three times a week. Some professional athletes and serious amateurs can even go to lower percentages and still be fine.

Athletes have to be considered as special cases when you talk about how fat affects health. This is because they can eat an ample and nutritious diet and still be thin. They're slender not because they undereat, but because they're very active physically.

Nonexercisers, on the other hand, can be thin only if they limit their calorie intake. This increases their chance of missing essential nutrients. If they do fail to get proper nutrition, they may be thin, but they won't be healthy.

Acceptable and Unacceptable Deviations

For all but the most dedicated athletes, the body-fat percentages of 20 to 25 percent for women, 10 to 15 percent for men, are the best ones for perfect health.

You don't need to panic if you're a few points off. In fact, you can be as much as 10 percentage points above the ideal for someone of your sex and activity level and still be in no real trouble. But as you deviate seriously on either side of the norms, you increase your chance of hurting your health. The greater the deviation, and the longer it persists, the greater the risk. In other words, the fatter you are, and the longer you're fat, the greater the danger to your health.

Let's leave aside for now the lower body-fat percentages that apply to vigorous exercisers and concentrate on the 25 and 15 percent norms for the average woman or man. After all, heavy exercisers are the people least likely to have weight problems.

If you're an average woman whose weight consists of 35 percent fat, or an average man whose weight is 25 percent fat, are you too fat?

Medically speaking, no. You may not like the way you look, and you may think you'd feel better if you got down to the ideal percentage. If so, fine. It certainly won't hurt you to lose a few pounds. But an upward deviation of 10 percent or less probably is not harming your health or curtailing your life span.

If you go higher, however, you're getting into the danger zone. The average woman whose fat makes up from 36 to 60 percent of her body weight is moderately obese, or moderately overweight. The same is true of the average man whose fat content is from 26 to 50 percent of his weight. In this category, excess fat is jeopardizing good health.

Fat percentages of more than 60 percent for women and 50 percent for men constitute gross or morbid obesity. This degree of overweight is life-threatening in an extreme and imminent way.

MEASURING YOUR FAT

We're making progress. Now at least you know what "fat" means. The next step is learning how to calculate how much of it you're carrying around.

Where to Look

You have fat tucked away in just about every part of your body. It's in your blood, bone marrow, muscles, liver, and spleen, and around your organs and glands.

But more than 50 percent of your fat is layered over your muscles and under your skin. This fat layer is attached to your skin. So the simplest way to measure body fat is to pinch some skin and see how much fat comes along with it. The thicker the skin fold, the fatter you are.

How to Measure Your Fat Content

The best way to measure skin-fold thickness is with a skin caliper. You can buy one at a medical supply house or sports equipment store, or you can order one from one of the firms listed on the next pages. A caliper can cost anywhere from about $8 to about $20.

The One-Pinch Test

This test is a quick and easy way to get an idea of where you stand in relation to your ideal body-fat percentage. All you do is tightly pinch the skin on the back of your upper arm, midway between the shoulder and the elbow. Measure the thickness of the fold with a caliper or ruler. If you are using a caliper, the result will be in *millimeters*. If you are using a ruler, the result will be in *inches*, measured in sixteenths of an inch. (Be sure to hold the ruler across the *top* of the skin fold you're measuring.)

In the table you will find skin-fold measurements for men and women, given both in sixteenths of an inch and in millimeters. Look at the number that is right for your sex and age. If your triceps skin-fold measurement is greater than the number given in the table, you have too much body fat.

MINIMUM TRICEPS SKIN-FOLD THICKNESS

AGE	MEN		WOMEN	
	16TH IN.	MILLIMETERS	16TH IN.	MILLIMETERS
18	10	15	17	27
19	10	15	17	27
20	10	16	17	28
21	11	17	17	28
22	12	18	17	28
23	12	18	17	28
24	13	19	17	28
25	13	20	18	29
26	13	20	18	29
27	14	21	18	29
28	14	22	18	29
29	15	23	18	29
30–50	15	23	20	30

Adapted from C. C. Seltzer and Jean Mayer, "A Simple Criterion of Obesity," *Postgraduate Medicine* 38 (August 1965): A-101–A-107.

Buying a Caliper

Several types of calipers are available. Here are three kinds; all are accurate and reasonably priced:

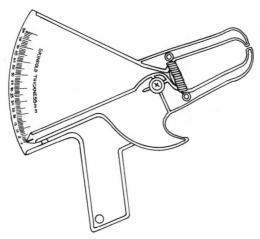

1. *Slimglide Caliper:* Large and impressive, made of plastic, accurate. Available in stores or from Sweat, P.O. Box 576, 3219 Close Court, Cincinnati, OH 45201, or from Creative Health Products, 5148 Saddle Ridge Road, Plymouth, MI 48170. $20

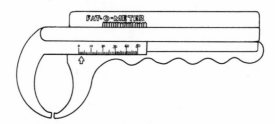

2. *Fat-o-Meter Caliper:* Accurate and smaller than the first. A little more difficult to use. Available in stores or from Health and Education Services, 80 Fairbanks, Unit 12, Addison, IL 60101. $9.95

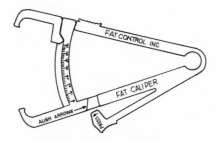

3. *Fat Control Caliper:* A very lightweight caliper that can be put in your pocket. No less accurate than the others. Available from stores or from Fat Control, P.O. Box 10117, Towson, MD 21204. $8.95

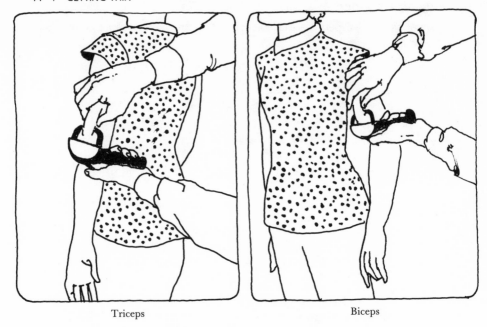

Triceps   Biceps

THESE FOUR AREAS TO BE MEASURED
FOR BODY-FAT DETERMINATION

The Four-Pinch Test

Fat patterns differ widely from person to person. Men and women deposit fat very differently. So do older people and younger ones. There are also individual variations in body build. Some people deposit fat mainly in their hips, others in their breasts, others in their bellies. By measuring in four different places, you will get a more accurate picture of your own body-fat percentage. In this case, you must use a skin caliper. You should measure the *triceps* (back of upper arm); the *biceps* (front of upper arm); the *suprailiac* (just above the hipbone at your side); and the *subscapular* (just below your shoulderblade in the back; you will need a wall mirror or a friend to help with this one). The pictures show you exactly how to make these measurements.

Write down the four measurements and add them up. Find the number you get — the sum of the four skin-fold measurements — on the

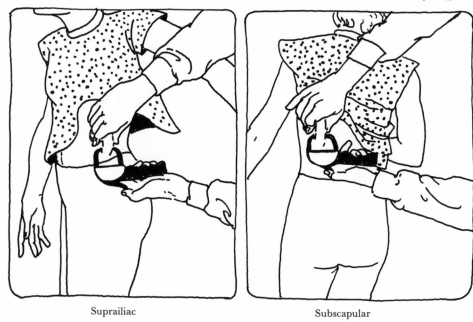

Suprailiac   Subscapular

table. Next to it, on the right, you will see two other columns: "Percent of body fat in women" and "Percent of body fat in men." *The number in the body-fat percentage column for your sex opposite the sum of your skin-fold measurements represents the percentage of body fat you are carrying.*

How To Use a Caliper

To measure skin thickness, grasp a one-inch length of skin (not more) over the recommended area between your thumb and index or middle finger. Take the skin caliper in your other hand and open the jaws. Place the open jaws horizontally to the group over the pinched skin. Then release the jaws so the spring will cause them to pinch the skin snugly. (The jaws should stop moving immediately — if they keep moving, you've pinched too much skin.) Read the skin thickness on the caliper gauge.

THE FOUR-PINCH TEST

SUM OF 4 SKIN FOLDS (IN MILLIMETERS)	PERCENT OF BODY FAT IN WOMEN	PERCENT OF BODY FAT IN MEN
25	18	12
30	20.5	13.5
35	23	15.5
40	24.5	17
50	28	20
55	29.5	21
60	30.5	22
65	32	23
70	33	24
75	34	25
80	35	25.5
85	36	26.5
90	36.5	27
95	37	28
100	38	28.5
105	39	29
115	40	30
125	41.5	31.5
135	42.5	32.5
145	44	33
160	45	34.5
180	47	36
200	49	37.5
220	50.5	38.5
250	52	40

FAT AND WEIGHT

Understandably, you may find it hard to break the habit of thinking in terms of weight instead of fat. You'll be happy to hear that you don't really have to. Now that you know your body-fat percentage, you can say something meaningful about ideal weight.

There's a formula for translating fat percentage into the more familiar terms of weight. It's based on the ideals of 15 percent body fat for men and 25 percent for women. (Remember to subtract 5 percent if you're a regular strenuous exerciser.) Here is the formula:

Present weight × (present body-fat % − ideal body-fat %) = weight to be lost.

For example, if you're a woman who weighs 130 pounds and you have 30 percent body fat, the formula for you looks like this:

(a) 30% − 25% (ideal body fat %) = 5% excess body fat.

(b) 130 lbs. (present weight) × .05 (5% excess body fat) = 6.5 lb.

In other words, you should lose 6.5 pounds in order to achieve an ideal weight of 123.5 pounds, and an ideal body-fat percentage of 25. If you're a man, the formula is the same. Just substitute 15 ideal body-fat percentage for 25. If you're a man who weighs 200 pounds, of which 25 percent is fat, you have 10 percent too much fat. Your perfect weight will be your 200 pounds *minus* the percentage of excess body fat:

(a) 25% − 15% (ideal body fat %) = 10% excess body fat.

(b) 200 lbs. (present weight) × .10 (10% excess fat) = 20 lbs.

Let me remind you again that there's a good deal of leeway between absolute perfection and a true weight problem. Your body-fat percentage can be up to 10 over the ideal before you're obese in any clinical sense. Within the 10 percent margin, losing weight is a matter of personal preference, not medical necessity.

When you look at it that way, chances are that you're not quite as "fat" as you thought you were. That should be a comfort, even if you're not entirely satisfied with your size. Keep it in mind as you go on to explore how people get fat, and why they often stay that way.

6.

HOW FAT
PEOPLE ARE DIFFERENT

IF you're a veteran in the war on fat, you've probably said it yourself a thousand times:

"I eat hardly anything, but I still can't lose weight."

Or,

"I'm overweight because I have a bad metabolism."

You've battled so hard and failed so often to get utterly and permanently sleek. It just hasn't worked. By now you have a sneaking suspicion that certain mysterious forces have conspired to make you "naturally" fat and other people "naturally" thin. You're looking for some innate difference between the pudgy you and the slender "them."

Your thin friends sneer skeptically. They assume you're gluttonous, paranoid, or just making excuses. In fact, you're none of these things. Not really.

FAT PEOPLE <u>ARE</u> PHYSIOLOGICALLY DIFFERENT

You're probably on the right track, though maybe for the wrong reasons. You're perfectly correct in observing that fat people and skinny people are different — very different. In several vital ways, their bodies don't function alike.

But you're wrong if you think that being different is what makes you fat. It's the other way around. *Being fat makes your body behave differently, in ways that tend to keep you fat.*

Calorie Intake and Output

You may be right in saying that you don't overeat. Scientists have demonstrated that active thin people generally take in an average of 600 calories a day *more* than fat people.

The difference is that the active skinnies are able to burn up many more calories with a high level of physical activity. They burn off their excess intake not just while they're exercising, but all the time. The fatties, on the other hand, keep squirreling away every extra calorie as fat.

Nothing can alter the basic equation that says if you take in more calories than you burn up, the excess ends up as fat. This is true for fat people and thin ones alike. But as you'll see in this chapter and the next, fat people often have faulty mechanisms governing either the output of energy, the intake of food, or both.

Even when they manage to lose weight by dieting, fatties usually find that the loss is dismally temporary. They never seem to lose the tendency to gain weight easily and take it off only with profound difficulty. They find that being thin through dieting alone means staying on a lifelong diet that would starve a gnat. It's little wonder that hardly anyone can manage to do it. Almost everybody who has ever lost weight through diet alone is familiar with the yo-yo syndrome, the dangerous and disappointing ricochet between loss and gain.

Metabolic Differences

Once again, blaming your weight problem on your metabolism is about half right. If you're fat, you probably do have a slow metabolism. But you're putting the cart before the horse once more. Your metabolism isn't doing it to you. You're doing it to it. You're sluggish because you're fat, not the other way around.

Metabolism is a much-abused term. What does it really mean?

Your metabolism is the whole complex of your body's functions. It's the sum of all the chemical reactions that go on in your body to make new tissue and produce energy. It's the total of processes by which your body uses fuel — the food you eat — to keep itself alive, intact, and functioning.

The chemical conversion of food to energy is a metabolic basic that is crucial to the question of whether you're fat or thin. How much food is used up for energy and for body growth and maintenance, and how much is stored as fat? How quickly and efficiently does your body burn its fuel supply?

Metabolic rates vary widely among individuals. If you're thin, your metabolism is a high-speed superjet, burning loads of calories. If you're fat, it's a lazy locomotive, chugging along with minimal energy output, using its fuel slowly and sparingly.

Later in the chapter you'll read about specific metabolic components that have great influence over whether you're fat or thin. For now, just remember this all-important fact: *A sluggish metabolism can be altered, primarily through exercise.* If you become more active and lose weight, your metabolism usually readjusts itself automatically to the change. Eventually, it should run at just as brisk a clip as that of the "naturally" slender person you envy.

EXERCISE: THE KEY

If you're a chronic dieter, you already know that diets generally promise more than they deliver. While an iron will and a good diet may be able to get you thin, you don't tend to stay that way.

One reason is that diets stress the wrong side of the thermodynamic equation governing weight loss. That equation says that you lose weight when you expend more calories than you take in.

Limiting calories is fine, as far as it goes. But it does nothing to maximize your body's capacity to burn calories. As a result, the best you can hope for from a diet is a temporarily thin body that's still shackled to a fat metabolism. Begin to eat normally, and the weight comes right back, often with interest.

This is worse than dispiriting; it's dangerous. Weight swings can shorten your life. Every time you gain weight rapidly you narrow your arteries with deposits of that fatty substance called plaque, which I discussed in Chapter 4. As you know, plaquing can lead to high blood pressure, strokes, and heart attacks.

Laboratory experiments demonstrate the point. In one study, doctors divided a litter of genetically fat rats into two groups. One group stayed fat. The other ate a diet manipulated to make the rats gain and lose weight. The rats that stayed fat lived a third longer than the ones that lost and regained.

Increasing Calorie Burnoff

Exercise, far more than diet, is the key to making you metabolically — and permanently — slender.

Many a diet guru has told you that exercise isn't important. They reason that if you have to walk seventeen miles to burn up a single pound of fat, why bother?

They're missing the point. Extra calories burned during exercise are only part of the story. What happens afterward is probably even more important. A metabolism revved up by a hard workout will stay in an elevated state for four to six hours after the workout is over, burning up additional calories.

Of course, the rate of burnoff during this period is not as fast as it is during the workout itself. It diminishes steadily. Still, the burnoff rate during the four to six hours after exercise is about 10 percent higher than it would be if you hadn't exercised.

Basal metabolism — the rate at which you burn calories while at rest — varies quite a bit from person to person. But a fairly common figure is 60 calories per hour. At this rate, you burn 360 calories in six hours of a sedentary day. But a strenuous workout would be followed by a burnoff of 396 calories in the same six hours.

The difference may not sound like much, but it mounts up. If you exercise hard for at least half an hour only three days a week, the increased post-workout burnoff can make a weight difference of 5 to 10 pounds in a year if there is no change in your diet.

As you'll see later in the chapter, it's also likely that strenuous exercise will cause you to burn more calories not only for a few hours after a workout, but all the time — even while you sleep.

It's no accident that athletes are seldom fat, or that chronically fat people are also chronically sedentary. Exercise, and exercise alone, has the capacity to recalibrate your metabolism to a "naturally" thin mode.

Storing Fat

Remember the camel, the seal, the bird, and the bear in Chapter 3? All have a remarkable ability to store massive amounts of fat. They stuff themselves, of course, but that's not their only technique.

About three weeks before the bird flies south, it becomes very inactive.

It does little else but eat. When the bear is about to hibernate, it becomes idle. When the seal prepares for the mating season, and the camel for a desert crossing, they become inactive.

Inactivity is a signal to store fat.

The principle works the same way in humans.

Since the current model of the human body dates back thousands of years, it's a body designed for physical activity. It is geared to hunt for food, not saunter to the microwave; to walk for miles, not push a gas pedal. It is meant for a life in which mere survival requires a lot of strenuous hustle.

Today this body, unchanged for centuries, is confronted with a world that has turned upside down in only a few generations. Your mind may be able to cope with future shock, but your body has no idea what to make of it.

Your body assumes from your inactivity that for some reason you need to store fat. Perhaps game is scarce or the crops have failed, and a famine is on the way. So it sets out to protect you the best way it knows how, by helping you store fat. Your metabolism slows down, and the pounds start piling up.

THE METABOLIC POWERHOUSES

The basic unit of metabolism is the cell. All your life, your body's trillions of living cells are constantly converting food to energy. How the energy is used depends on the organ or the anatomical system or structure to which particular cells belong.

For instance, the energy can go into making your heart beat, your lungs breathe, your brain think, your muscles move, and your digestive system break down food. All these activities are metabolic processes in which energy is produced and consumed. All go on at varying speeds, depending on the individual's own metabolic rate.

But scientists have pinpointed three particular metabolic mechanisms as being especially important in determining why some people are fatter than others. They are:

- Brown fat
- The sodium-potassium pump
- Hormones

All three figure prominently in how quickly and efficiently calories are burned. And it appears that all three are less efficient in people who are overweight and sedentary than in people who are thin and active.

Brown Fat

There are two kinds of fat in your body. The only kind I've discussed so far is yellow fat — so called because yellow is the natural color of fat.

Yellow fat is the kind you store in your fat cells and mobilize for energy as needed. It is the fat that's located in many parts of your body and is most evident just beneath your skin. This is the fat that can be a friend or an enemy, depending on whether you have the right amount or too much. If you're trying to lose weight, this yellow fat is the fat you're trying to get rid of.

Brown fat is a different matter altogether. It is called "brown" because it has a rich, dense supply of blood vessels. Scientists have noted its distinctive color in work on animals and with human infants. The amount present in human adults is so small that it cannot be seen and researchers have had to study it mainly by observing the way it behaves, rather than by looking at it directly.

The traditional way to study brown-fat activity was to measure the heat it produced. However, just lately scientists have been able to use a technique called "surface thermography" that translates varying heat patterns into visual images. In this way, they've been able to locate heat patterns in just those places where we would expect to find brown fat. This has also allowed them to observe its behavior with more precision than in earlier studies.

Unlike your vast store of yellow fat, your tiny supply of brown fat is not distributed throughout your body, nor can it move from place to place. The brown fat is very localized and it stays put because it has a very specific primary purpose.

BROWN FAT'S FUNCTION

As you know, yellow fat offers a bounty of gifts: it can provide portable food, water, energy, warmth, and brain sustenance, and it promotes female fertility.

Brown fat, on the other hand, is in your body for one main reason: to warm your vital internal organs, especially your heart.

Brown fat is located between your shoulderblades, under your armpits, around your kidneys, and around all the large veins and arteries near your heart. Its strategic placement allows it to warm cold blood moving toward the heart so that the heart won't be chilled. If it weren't for brown fat, blood reaching the heart unheated could cause irregular heartbeats.

BROWN FAT AND CALORIES

To do its job, brown fat must be able to generate prodigious amounts of heat. It always does, though the exact amount varies among individuals.

The fuel used to produce this heat is yellow fat. Both brown-fat cells and yellow-fat cells contain yellow fat. The big difference is that yellow-fat cells only store the fuel; brown-fat cells burn it.

As you know, yellow fat has to move out of its storage cells before it can be burned to produce energy and heat. The fat cells that store it can't burn it themselves. Rather, they yield it into the bloodstream for transport to other cells — including brown-fat cells — that have the capacity to burn it. Until it's mobilized, the yellow fat produces virtually no energy on its own. It's mostly dead weight, useless as a calorie burner.

But the radically different brown fat is as active as the stored yellow fat is inert. In constantly consuming fuel and producing heat, brown fat requires and expends an enormous load of calories.

Exactly how many calories brown fat can dispose of is a highly variable matter, as you're about to see. But as a rule, the brown fat of thin and active people works harder and consumes significantly more calories than the brown fat of people who are obese and inactive. If you're one of those very active people, it may be possible for your brown fat to burn *all* the excess calories you eat.

BROWN-FAT RESPONSIVENESS

Your yellow-fat tissue can grow or shrink as you gain or lose weight. This is not true of brown fat. Brown fat ordinarily makes up only about 1 percent of your total body fat, and weight fluctuations do nothing to increase or decrease it.

However, brown fat does grow or diminish, and it becomes more or less active, in response to other factors. These factors are:

- Cold
- Eating
- Exercise

The reason for increased brown-fat activity in response to cold is obvious. The tissue has to work harder to maintain the internal heat you need to protect your heart.

But along with its prime function as a thermostat, brown fat seems to have a secondary role as an internal safeguard against excessive weight gain. The more you overeat, the harder the brown fat works to consume the excess.

When it comes to exercise, brown fat seems to follow the evolutionary logic that equates inactivity with fat storage. If you're inactive, the brown fat burns calories sluggishly. But when you're very active, the brown fat assumes you have no need for a great amount of stored fat, and it sets about burning off some of the excess.

Some scientists believe there is a genetic component that helps determine how active your brown fat will be. This question is still unsettled. But we know that the heredity factor, if any, is far less important a determinant than cold, eating, and exercise.

NORADRENALINE

The messenger that tells the brown fat what size and activity level to attain is a hormone called *noradrenaline* or *norepinephrine*. Noradrenaline is a natural stimulant produced by the adrenal glands near your kidneys and by nerve cells.

When you're subjected to cold, or when you eat or exercise, your brain sends out impulses along a nerve network, prompting the adrenal glands to step up production of noradrenaline.

Hard exercise can cause noradrenaline to rise to five times its normal level in your bloodstream. The amount of increase in response to cold depends on the degree of cold and how long you're exposed to it. Similarly, noradrenaline increases brought on by eating vary according to the amount and frequency of food intake. The more you eat, the higher the level. The more often you eat, the longer the level stays high.

As cold, eating, and exercise prompt the increased production of noradrenaline, they also make your brown fat more sensitive to the hormone. This is another factor that causes the brown fat to enlarge and become more active.

BROWN FAT AND COLD

If you're exposed to cold weather for only half an hour each day, within two weeks your brown fat will enlarge and become more active.

The extent to which cold stimulates brown-fat activity and size varies according to how cold it is and how long your exposure to it lasts. But researchers have demonstrated that the activity can increase as much as 10 to 20 percent above normal.

I hope you don't infer from this that I recommend your standing barefoot in the snow in order to rev up your brown fat. Improving your eating and activity habits will be far more productive.

BROWN FAT AND EATING

In theory, if you take in 3,500 calories in excess of what you need for body maintenance and energy, you should gain one pound of fat. Actually, you don't.

Many scientists believe that the reason you don't is that brown fat, stimulated by eating, burns off some, or even all, of the excess. It is estimated that very energetic brown fat can dispose of all 3,500 calories that would otherwise end up as a pound of fat — and then some.

In fact, quite a number of reputable studies at universities in the United States and England have reported finding some very active people who took in from 5,000 to 7,000 extra calories *a day* without gaining weight! And at one Vermont prison, an experiment with inmate volunteers to study weight-gain patterns found that systematically overfeeding and exercising prisoners to the same degree produced massive weight gains in some but very little in others. In all these studies, researchers attributed the disposal of the excess weight to very active brown fat.

These results are astonishing. Humans generally need around 2,000 to 2,500 calories a day for basic maintenance. Most of us would be hard put just to eat two to three times that much, much less burn it off. Needless to say, individuals who manage such a feat are rare exceptions, not the rule. But they do serve as indicators of the enormous calorie-burning power of brown fat.

The degree of, and length of increase in, brown-fat activity after a meal depend mostly on the size of the meal. The bigger the meal, the greater the production of heat in response to it, and the longer the response lasts. A real feast can increase brown fat's heat production by a factor of 10 to 20 percent above normal, with the speedup extending as long as six hours.

But this is not an argument for confining your eating to one big meal a day. On the contrary, getting a big brown-fat response is less important than prolonging a smaller response. In other words, eating numerous small meals causes a greater calorie burnoff in the long run than eating a few large ones.

This is one reason why nibblers are better at maintaining their weight than gorgers. The nibblers can keep their brown fat working hard almost perpetually.

The lesson here is that five or six small meals a day can keep your brown-fat activity elevated for almost all your waking hours.

BROWN FAT AND EXERCISE

Scientists know less about the relationship between exercise and brown fat than they do about the tissue's response to cold and to eating.

But there is a very credible theory that brown fat does respond to exercise by consuming more calories for four to six hours after a hard workout. Researchers have established that there is a rise in body heat during the post-exercise period. The rise is greater than what can be accounted for by the obvious metabolic speedups associated with exercise — increased heart rate, muscular activity, and the like.

This increased heat has been attributed by some investigators to brown-fat response. Brown fat cannot be observed directly. But heat sensors placed on the body during the post-workout period have recorded elevated heat levels over the areas where brown fat is located. Scientists theorize that this increase may be in response to a temporary increase in noradrenaline levels brought on by exercise. The noradrenaline increase, which may be as much as five times the normal level, dissipates in about an hour. Nonetheless, the reasoning goes, this temporary buildup may be enough to account for the longer-lasting rise in body heat — just as when you turn off the gas flame in an oven, the oven walls continue to generate heat for some time afterward.

There is a second exercise-related theory that has even wider support. This one holds that aside from its possible ability to stimulate brown fat on its own, exercise exaggerates the stimulating effects of cold and eating. In other words, a very active person will have a greater brown-fat response than a sedentary person when he or she eats or is exposed to cold, just because of exercising.

There are many specifics about brown fat that require more study, and in fact the subject is getting a lot of attention from researchers these days. But despite gaps in our knowledge, it seems clear that encouraging brown-fat activity with good exercise and eating habits can have a significant bearing on weight control.

The Sodium Pump

In examining how brown fat works, you begin to see a pattern that appears to hold true for all the metabolic factors that help govern your weight: whether you're active and thin, or sedentary and fat, you're in a metabolic cycle that tends to perpetuate itself.

The more active you are, the better your metabolism works to keep you thin by expending excess calories. The more sedentary you are, the more likely your metabolism is to keep you fat. Your body, requiring only a low-level energy output, encourages you to store more calories as fat.

Some respected research indicates that this rule applies to a complicated metabolic mechanism called the *sodium-potassium pump,* or sodium pump for short.

THE HUMAN ELECTRICAL SYSTEM

The human body is the world's most complex electrical system. Every time you see, think, run, talk, digest food, or experience any other life function, you're able to do it because electrical impulses are at work. Electrical messages tell your heart when to beat, your bowels when to move, your brain when to register pain.

To understand how this works, think of your body's trillions of living cells as tiny batteries. Like all batteries, they work by passing an electrical impulse between different concentrations of minerals.

In the case of the cells, the main minerals involved are sodium and potassium. Both minerals are present in your body all the time in the fluid bathing your cells and in the fluid inside the cells. The natural tendency would be for the minerals to be at the same concentration both inside and outside the cells. But if this were the case, there would be no electrical conduction.

Conduction takes place because the sodium pump works every second of every day to pump sodium out from inside the cells and to draw potassium from the outside in. Thus you always have more sodium on the outside and more potassium on the inside, and electrical impulses can pass from one area to another.

HOW THE PUMP WORKS

"Sodium pump" is a convenient name for this rearranger of minerals, but it isn't really a very good one. It's a highly misleading metaphor.

In fact, you don't have just one sodium pump. You have quadrillions of sodium pumps, spread throughout your body.

Each of your cells is something like a balloon filled with water. The balloon itself, the outside of the cell, is called the cell membrane. Each membrane has thousands of tiny holes, or pores, through which the minerals pass back and forth. And each pore has its own sodium pump.

Every little sodium pump is a sort of combination gatekeeper, maitre d', and bouncer. It checks minerals outside the cell to identify them. If the mineral is potassium, it gets invited in. If it's sodium, the door is barred. Meanwhile, the pump keeps watch on minerals inside the cell. When it spots sodium, the sodium gets booted out.

The word *pump* is misleading in itself. Actually, scientists don't yet know the exact mechanics by which the cell membrane redistributes minerals. No true "pumping" has ever been observed. They do know, however, that the cell membranes move in some mysterious way that forces minerals to concentrate in the proper places to allow electrical conduction.

They also know that the sodium pump is essential to organic life. If your sodium-pump system stopped working even for a few seconds, sodium would leak inside your cells and potassium would leak out. Electrical activity would stop, and you'd die instantly.

CALORIES: SODIUM PUMP VS. BROWN FAT

Your brown fat and your sodium pump are both calorie burners, but they have little else in common. Don't confuse the two.

As you saw, brown fat consumes calories by burning yellow fat to produce heat. Something very different goes on with the sodium pump.

Obviously, it takes a lot of energy, or calories, to keep trillions of cell membranes in constant motion policing mineral concentrations. But in this case, the energy has nothing to do with the burning of yellow fat. Rather, it involves a complicated interplay between the burning of sugar inside the cell, and chemical activity taking place in the cell membrane.

Each membrane contains a chemical called *adenosine triphosphate*, or ATP. ATP constantly releases energy. It is always breaking down and then rebuilding itself with the help of other chemicals. Both processes release energy. The rebuilding process is fueled by sugar metabolism inside the cell. The sugar metabolism needed by the sodium pump to rebuild ATP is what accounts for its calorie-consuming capacity.

Considerable controversy surrounds the question of how the sodium pump stacks up against brown fat as a calorie burner. Some scientists give brown fat the edge, contending it can burn off all the excess calorie intake in some very active people.

But theoretically, at least, the sodium pump might have an even greater capacity. While brown fat makes up only a tiny part of your body, the sodium pump involves every single living cell. And while brown-fat activity has peaks and valleys in response to outside stimuli, the sodium pump has to work all the time.

Of course, whether the sodium pump works at the same *level* in all people all the time is another matter.

THE SODIUM PUMP AND EXERCISE

The chief proponent of the sodium pump's calorie-burning capacity is the highly esteemed scientist George L. Blackburn. Dr. Blackburn is associate professor of surgery at Harvard Medical School and one of America's leading obesity specialists.

He contends that the sodium-pump system operates with much greater efficiency in thin, active people than in people who are overweight and inactive. He has done research showing that fat, sedentary people have sodium pumps that are 22 percent less active than those of thinner people who exercise often. This means the calorie-burning capacity of the pump is 22 percent lower in the fatter people. Expressed another way, it means the pumps on their cell membranes work 22 percent less hard.

On the optimistic side, Dr. Blackburn also demonstrated that exercise can bring sluggish sodium pumps up to par. Measuring sodium-pump activity in terms of energy consumption in red blood cells, he tested overweight people before and after putting them on an exercise program. After they began exercising regularly, the test subjects showed a 22 percent increase in sodium-pump activity.

THE SODIUM-PUMP CONTROVERSY

In the last few years, Dr. Blackburn's findings have been disputed by some scientists in America and Europe. There is some basic disagreement over whether the sodium pump is, in fact, more active in thin people. For example, Dr. George Bray, a professor of medicine at UCLA, does not agree with the sodium-pump theory of Dr. Blackburn. He has shown that the livers of skinny people do not have more active sodium pumps than those of obese people.

Nevertheless, Dr. Blackburn remains the premier researcher in this particular area, and he stands staunchly by his theory. Moreover, he has an impressive amount of evidence to back him up, and his arguments are more persuasive than those of his critics so far.

Like brown fat, the sodium pump holds some mysteries as yet unsolved. More work needs to be done to quantify the sodium pump's precise calorie-burning potential. We need to find exactly why the sodium-pump activity changes with a person's weight and exercise level. We need to gauge the effect, if any, of heredity on sodium-pump activity.

For now, however, most scientists believe with Dr. Blackburn that the sodium pump does have great impact on determining and regulating weight. It behaves most efficiently in people who are physically active, and this high efficiency is a major factor in keeping exercisers thin.

Exercise burns excess calories in and of itself. Brown-fat response may keep calorie burnoff high for four to six hours after exercise. But it's the sodium pump that appears to help regular exercisers burn more calories around the clock, even while they sleep.

Hormones

Brown fat and the sodium pump are calorie burners themselves, and as such they're important in determining how fat or thin you may be.

Hormones are different. Their importance lies not with their own calorie-burning capacity, but with their role in directing energy consumption, expenditure, and storage in the rest of the body.

Most hormones have more than one function, and several of them figure in controlling your weight. When people blame obesity on a "glandular problem," it's these hormones they're talking about — usually inaccurately. True glandular obesity is very rare, making up only about 1 percent of all obesity cases.

It's true that thin, active people tend to have better hormone functions than fat people. But here again, malfunctioning hormones are usually the *result* of being fat, not the cause. And the malfunctions are almost always correctable through weight loss and stepped-up exercise.

HORMONE MULTIFUNCTIONS
Hormones would be a lot easier to explain if they weren't so versatile. Unfortunately, their ability to do so many different things makes them hard to pigeonhole.

Some hormones encourage you to store fat, others to mobilize it for energy. These hormones properly belong in a discussion of metabolism, or calorie output. But some of these same hormones also have a bearing on appetite, or calorie intake. Take noradrenaline, for example. Along with helping you burn more calories, it can also help curb your hunger.

For the sake of convenience, this chapter will deal mainly with how hormones help or hinder energy output. In the next chapter, you'll meet some of these same hormones, along with some altogether new ones, in their guise as influencers of appetite.

INSULIN

Insulin is the most powerful of the pro-fat hormones and the biggest promoter of fat storage. You learned a little in Chapter 4 about insulin abnormalities in fat people. Now for some details on how and why this hormone works the way it does.

You'll remember that insulin's main job is to reduce blood levels of fat and sugar. It drives the substances out of your bloodstream and into your cells. As you'll see, it not only performs this task, but does it in a way that assures a maximum accumulation of body fat. Evolution helps explain why.

Insulin is a holdover from those distant days when it was an advantage to be able to store as much fat as possible. Body fat meant survival in lean times. Insulin works to conserve your fat stores by striving to make your body use sugar for energy instead of fat.

It does this in three main ways:
- It drives fat into fat cells for storage.
- It drives sugar into cells for fuel or storage.
- It causes your liver to convert sugar to fat at an accelerated rate.

Insulin and Fat The fat in your bloodstream can come from three sources: the fatty food you eat, fat stores released from your fat cells, and fat stores released from your liver.

Some of your cells pick up this circulating fat and burn it for energy. Most of the rest is herded into your fat cells by insulin.

The insulin acts directly on fat-cell membranes, binding to them in a way that forces the fat inside and prevents its escape back into the bloodstream. In other words, insulin tries to see to it that all the fat it can round up gets stored and stays stored.

You'll recall that when you're low on sugar, perhaps because you're dieting, your body calls out fat from your fat cells to burn for energy. Insulin fights this process and can disrupt it.

This is one reason why a dieter who lapses and has one big meal may note with dismay that weight loss stops for a while, even if he or she goes right back on the diet. A big meal brings on a big insulin response. And at high levels the insulin is able for a time to keep fat trapped in its storage cells. The fat stays put, despite the efforts of opposing chemical forces to dislodge it.

How your body responds to insulin depends on how many insulin receptors you have. Insulin receptors are special formations on the outer membranes of many of your cells. The insulin attaches to these structures and is carried into the cells by them. The more insulin receptors you have, the more sensitive you are to the hormone and the less of it your body requires. The less insulin you have, the less likely you are to be fat. So increasing the number of receptors helps keep you slim.

Research shows that you can increase the number of receptors by reducing your body fat, exercising, eating less fatty food, and eating more high-fiber food. (As you'll learn in Chapter 11, high-fiber food consists of the complex carbohydrates found mostly in fruits, vegetables, and grains.)

Insulin and Sugar Most of the food you eat gets into your bloodstream in the form of sugar, not fat. So sugar is your body's best indicator of whether your environment is supplying you with enough food. This is probably why sugar, not fat, is the trigger for insulin response. The hormone responds to blood levels of sugar, the more reliable indicator, even though it acts on both sugar and fat.

The sugar we're talking about here is glucose, or blood sugar. Most of your food is converted by your digestive system to glucose, which is the only type of sugar that circulates throughout your bloodstream.

Insulin drives glucose into cells the same way it forces in the fat, by binding to cell membranes.

The amount of glucose in your blood depends on when, what, and how much you've eaten. As soon as you eat, your glucose level rises. If the meal is a big one, and especially if it's rich in carbohydrates, the glucose level will become very high.

At a certain point, which varies from person to person, the glucose rise prompts the pancreas to release insulin to clear away the excess glucose. The higher the glucose level, the greater the insulin flow.

As the insulin does its work, the glucose level falls. Once it gets low enough, you start to feel hungry again.

Thin people tend to maintain their sugar-insulin interplay on a fairly even keel. This way there are no steep hills and deep valleys as the two substances alternate their rise and fall in the bloodstream.

But, as you know, fat people react differently. You've already seen how overfull fat cells make you resistant to insulin. But this is only one problem. Another is that fat people have higher thresholds for triggering insulin release. For some unknown reason, they have to eat more before the insulin starts flowing. And once it does respond, the insulin flows in abnormally large amounts.

One result is that more insulin courses through the blood to force both sugar and fat into the cells. A second result is that the insulin surge makes the glucose level take a steep and sudden plunge, and the person is hungry again.

Sugar Storage and Conversion Most of the cells that pick up glucose from your bloodstream can burn it for immediate energy. But cells in your muscles and in your liver have an option. They can either burn it or store it. In its stored form, the glucose is called *glycogen.*

You'll remember from Chapter 3 that unlike fat, glycogen can be stored only in small amounts. The muscles take in only what they can hold, and they must deplete their store by burning it for energy before they can accept any more.

The liver doesn't have much storage capacity for glycogen either. But unlike the muscles, the liver can accumulate and deal with a surplus of sugar.

If more sugar is available than can be stored as glycogen, the liver has two choices. It can get rid of some existing glycogen by reconverting it to glucose and sending it back into the bloodstream to supply energy. Or it can convert some glycogen to fat and route it to the fat cells for storage. The result? More body fat.

Of course, insulin encourages the liver to choose the fat-storing alternative. It does this by helping chemicals called *enzymes* convert the glycogen to fat.

Nibbling vs. Gorging Along with brown fat, insulin offers an argument for controlling your weight by eating small, frequent meals. A small meal brings on a small insulin response. Frequent meals help keep glucose and insulin levels balanced and steady.

Keeping insulin levels low helps thwart the hormone's power to prompt fat storage and speed the conversion of sugar to fat. Maintaining a stable balance between glucose and insulin helps you avoid the glucose nosedives that bring on hunger.

Remember, insulin wasn't designed for the kind of life most modern Americans live. It was designed to help assure survival for our caveman ancestors, who tended to eat big rather than eat often. They sometimes hunted for days with no luck. But they gorged themselves once they made a kill. Insulin helped them make the most of large, infrequent meals.

CORTISOL

Cortisol is another pro-fat hormone. It leads to fat deposits, particularly on your trunk.

Cortisol is produced by your two adrenal glands. Fat people tend to produce more cortisol than thin people and eliminate it faster, too. Its role in fat storage isn't completely understood.

NORADRENALINE

You're already acquainted with noradrenaline, the important antifat hormone produced by your nerve cells and your adrenal glands. This is the messenger that prompts your brown fat to work harder and burn more calories. In addition, noradrenaline helps draw fat out of fat cells and make it available for burning.

As you know, thin people usually respond more to noradrenaline than fat people do. Again, this response can be improved by losing weight.

ADRENALINE

Adrenaline is another antifat hormone manufactured by the adrenal glands. A chemical cousin of noradrenaline, adrenaline is a very powerful fat mobilizer and prompter of high energy consumption.

THYROID HORMONES

Thyroid hormones are antifat hormones produced by the thyroid gland in your neck. They are also fat mobilizers, helping to release fat into your bloodstream and speed your metabolism.

Overeating can increase your body's production of thyroid hormones, and undereating can decrease it. Some people have taken thyroid hormones to help them lose weight. However, thyroid hormones should not be given to obese people with normally functioning thyroid glands because they cause loss of muscle tissue, rather than just fat. An underactive thyroid gland is a very rare cause of obesity.

Fat people have not been shown to have abnormal amounts of or responses to thyroid hormones.

GROWTH HORMONE

Growth hormone — this is its actual name — is antifat. One of its functions is to encourage the breakdown and burnoff of fat. In addition, it helps regulate your level of energy. Growth hormone is produced by a gland in your brain called the pituitary.

Fat people produce less growth hormone than thin people do in response to stress, exercise, sleep, and lower blood sugar levels. Weight loss improves this response.

ESTROGEN, PROGESTERONE, AND TESTOSTERONE

These are the major sex hormones. Estrogen and progesterone are primarily female hormones, testosterone primarily a male one. Estrogen is produced in many parts of your body, including your fat tissue. All three can promote weight gain. You'll find out more about them in Chapter 9, "The Fatter Sex."

HORMONES AND EXERCISE

Exercise causes changes in many hormone levels. In some cases, the alterations are brief, occurring only during the activity itself. Other changes are gradual or even permanent, lasting long after the exercise has ended.

Additional hormone changes can result from the weight loss that follows exercise. Exercise can also make your body more responsive to certain hormones, such as insulin, for example. Thus diabetics require less insulin when they exercise regularly.

FROM OUTPUT TO INTAKE

This chapter may have seemed pretty complicated in spots, but take heart. By now you probably know as much as many doctors do about the output side of the weight equation — the hows and whys of calorie burning.

But in emphasizing output, I'm not suggesting that you forget about diet altogether. Calorie intake is important. Not all fat people overeat, but overeating can certainly make you fat.

In the next chapter, you'll learn more about how your appetite works. In the process, you'll find another good argument for why you need to exercise.

7.

MORE DIFFERENCES: HOW APPETITE WORKS

IF bodies were banks and calories were cash, fat people would be rich. They're always making more deposits than withdrawals.

This certainly does not mean that all fat people are piggish overeaters. You saw in the last chapter how a fat person can eat less than a thin one and still maintain, and even increase, surplus fat. The difference is that the thin person is a big spender, while the fat one hoards calories.

Remember, when it comes to calories it's not the actual size of the deposit, or the size of the withdrawal, that matters. It's the balance between the two. If you put in more than you take out, you gain weight. If deposits and withdrawals match, you maintain weight. And if you take out more than you put in, you lose weight.

Underactivity is often responsible for giving fat people a calorie surplus. But what if you're one of those people who truly does overeat? Can you forget about exercise and just diet yourself into a calorie deficit?

Not likely.

You can't battle your appetite forever with much hope of winning. You have to find a way to make it work with you if you're to achieve and maintain a healthy weight. And this brings you right back to exercise. Exercise not only helps you spend more calories, it helps you deposit fewer. *Exercise is your best hope for curbing your appetite permanently.*

To understand why, you need to know more about how your appetite functions.

THEORIES OF HUNGER

In discussing the mechanics of appetite, I have to talk a lot about theories. Hard facts are in short supply. With all we've yet to learn about metabolism, we still know more about how our bodies use food than about why we eat in the first place. In many ways, hunger is an abiding mystery.

Obviously, we eat because we need food to live. But how does the body recognize, register, and regulate the need for food? In short, how do we get hungry?

It appears that hunger results from several contributing factors rather than from a single cause. But we know that hunger's master switch, its immediate trigger, lies in the brain. Let's start with that solid fact.

Your Appestat

There's a portion of the brain about the size and shape of a small clam-shell located dead center in your brain. It produces hormones, and is called the *hypothalamus*. We can think of it as a gland. It's relatively small in size, but enormous in power and complexity.

Like most glands, the hypothalamus appears to have a number of different functions. Researchers have found that one of these functions is somehow to govern appetite. The part of the hypothalamus that does this has therefore been dubbed the "appestat." It tells you when you're hungry and when you're full.

Thin people seem to have very efficient hypothalami. They know when they need food and when they've had enough, and they eat accordingly. But fat people often have glands that are faulty in some way. The signals they send out are too weak to govern appetite reliably.

The fault may lie with the gland itself. Or it may lie with substandard input from outside the brain. Here we arrive at those contributing causes for hunger that I mentioned. The hypothalamus triggers hunger. But what triggers the trigger?

GLUCOSE

Most scientists believe that the most important stimulus for prompting the hypothalamus to signal hunger has something to do with glucose.

There is evidence for theories that you get hungry when glucose levels drop in your blood, liver, pancreas, stomach, intestines, or several other sites.

But by far the best educated guess is that hunger begins when the glucose supply to your brain gets low. The hypothalamus senses an impending food deficit and begins sending out hunger messages. Your body responds in a variety of ways. You usually start to think about food, and your digestive system steps up secretions to help assimilate a coming meal.

STOMACH CONTRACTIONS AND STOMACH ACID

Most dieters are familiar with a growling stomach, and with the "sour" stomach they may sense if they go too long without eating.

Increased stomach contractions accompany hunger. There is also a rise in stomach levels of hydrochloric acid, which helps break down food. Some researchers believe that these two events are signals, or contributing causes, of hunger. It appears more likely, however, that they are results. In other words, it's probable that the stomach contracts and the acid builds up in response to directions from the hypothalamus.

SEROTONIN

Much of today's promising research on the chemistry of obesity is directed at a chemical called *serotonin*. Serotonin is a "neurotransmitter." This means it helps pass electrical messages along your nervous system and to your muscles.

You know that your brain sends messages to the rest of your body in the form of electrical impulses. When such an impulse reaches the end of a certain kind of nerve, the nerve end secretes serotonin. The serotonin forms a bridge to pass the impulse on to the next nerve, or to a muscle.

Serotonin is secreted by nerves throughout your body. It occurs in very high levels in your intestines. It can also be picked up by your bloodstream and carried from place to place.

Research has established a strong link between serotonin and hunger. Though we've yet to learn why, low levels of serotonin in the brain are associated with feelings of hunger. High brain levels inhibit hunger and make you feel full. Serotonin seems able to influence the hypothalamus in a rather direct way.

Serotonin levels depend in part on the kind of food you eat. Carbohydrates do more than any other food to keep the chemical at high levels in the brain.

CORTISOL

You'll remember cortisol from the last chapter as a hormone that promotes fat storage. It also promotes hunger.

Cortisol seems to act on the hypothalamus in some unknown way to signal hunger. It also figures in increasing the level of hydrochloric acid in the stomach.

ENDORPHINS

Endorphins are hormones manufactured by your brain. These morphinelike compounds are useful as natural pain blockers. But they have the unfortunate side effect of making you hungry. We don't know why. We do know that fat animals tend to have high endorphin levels.

In experiments with animals, scientists have found that blocking endorphins with chemicals can kill the appetite. But don't wait for antiendorphins to turn up on your druggist's shelf as miracle diet pills. Their side effects range from drowsiness to psychosis.

NORADRENALINE, ADRENALINE, AND DOPAMINE

Try to remember the last time you were enraged or terrified. Probably your entire attention was riveted on the object of your anger or fear. But had you been able to detach yourself and take a dispassionate reading of your body, you would have noticed that you weren't hungry. It's virtually impossible to feel hunger while in the grip of such strong emotion.

Like all animals, humans are equipped by nature with mechanisms for self-protection. When you're faced with a threat, your body reacts by flooding your system with certain hormones designed to help you fight or run.

They stimulate your brain so that you feel more alert. They rev up your heartbeat and respiration. They draw blood away from your skin and direct it toward your vital organs and toward your muscles, priming them for action.

While the hormones are stimulating body systems that can help you face danger, they're depressing systems that can't. Part of the process involves curtailing the flow of blood to the intestines, and alerting the hypothalamus in some way to switch off hunger signals.

The reason for this is obvious. When threatened, you don't sit down and eat before escaping or defending yourself.

The main hormones directing your "fight or flee" responses are noradrenaline, adrenaline, and dopamine. All are natural stimulants. You'll remember from the last chapter that adrenaline and noradrenaline are both antifat hormones produced by your adrenal glands and nerves.

Their ability to help you mobilize and burn fat is one of several contributions they make toward protecting you in a crisis.

Dopamine is produced by your body's nerve tissue. It, too, is a stimulant, behaving much the same way as noradrenaline.

Hunger and Exercise

Now we come to some of the reasons why exercise helps control your appetite.

You may be laboring under the misapprehension that exercising more will make you want to eat more. In fact, the opposite is the case for most people. It's true that heavy training — the sort that would daunt an Olympic athlete — increases the body's need for calories, and there's usually a proportionate increase in hunger.

But ordinary exercise — the regular, strenuous workouts that I recommend — makes you less hungry, not more.

Let's review some of the factors that scientists believe inhibit hunger:
- High levels of glucose, probably in the brain
- High brain levels of serotonin
- High blood levels of noradrenaline, adrenaline, and dopamine

Strenuous exercise tends to raise the levels of all these substances.

Exercise stimulates the liver to increase its release of stored glucose. As a result, more glucose circulates in your blood and is available to nourish your brain. The hypothalamus perceives the high glucose level, and you don't feel hungry.

In a similar way, exercise sets in motion a complex series of chemical changes that stimulate your production of serotonin. With high levels of serotonin in your brain, you feel less hungry.

Exercise can raise noradrenaline to five times its normal level in your blood, as you learned in the last chapter. In addition, it can increase adrenaline levels to two or three times the normal level. Again, by raising levels of antihunger chemicals, you inhibit your appetite.

The length of appetite suppression varies from chemical to chemical and from person to person. In general, though, you might expect to feel less hungry for as long as six hours after a hard workout.

Along with raising the levels of chemicals that diminish hunger, exercise tends to lower the levels of chemicals that promote it. Fat people tend to have abnormally high levels of cortisol and endorphins. Regular exercise has been shown to bring the levels into line with those of slimmer people.

THEORIES OF SATIETY

Of course, the most obvious way not to feel hungry is to feel full, and you feel full when you eat. This is true enough, but again, not as simple as it sounds. In fact, the way your appestat registers satiety, or fullness, is just as complicated as the way it registers hunger. And as with hunger, fullness seems to result from several causes instead of just one.

Here are the major theories about what makes you feel full:

Insulin Levels

The prevailing satiety theory is that your hypothalamus calls a halt to eating once insulin reaches a certain level in your spinal fluid. Spinal fluid is a liquid that circulates inside your spinal cord and brain.

As you know, high blood-glucose levels brought on by eating prompt the release of insulin. Insulin levels may be high in your bloodstream shortly after you start eating. But insulin filters very slowly from the blood into the spinal fluid. For most people, this means that it takes about twenty minutes from the onset of eating for feelings of fullness to begin.

We don't know exactly how the high levels of insulin in the spinal fluid make the hypothalamus signal fullness. But the effect itself has been observed in several experiments with animals. For instance, studies show that baboons stop eating once insulin levels rise in their spinal fluid.

No such studies have been done on humans, mainly because of physical difficulties involved in measuring brain insulin levels. But there's no reason to believe that our brains register fullness much differently from those of our primate cousins.

While we lack direct data on human brain insulin levels, we have many studies on insulin levels in the human bloodstream. We know from these that insulin usually enters the bloodstream of a fat person more slowly than it does a thin one. And we can infer from this that insulin is also tardy in reaching a fat person's spinal fluid.

Eat Dessert First

The best way to raise insulin levels in your brain is to raise your blood-sugar level. That's why it's a good idea to eat your dessert before you start the main portion of your meal. It will take at least twenty minutes for the insulin levels in your brain to rise so that you will feel full. Foods, such as fruit, that contain sugar will make you feel full sooner.

This assumption squares with the fact that some fat people eat more and eat longer than thin people before they begin to feel full. The greater intake indicates a lag time before insulin levels rise high enough in the spinal fluid to stimulate the appestat's satiety trigger.

The apparent link between insulin and satiety explains why weight-control specialists tell you to eat slowly. A leisurely meal prevents you from stuffing yourself before the insulin control apparatus has a chance to work.

Cholecystokinin

A relatively new satiety theory that's getting a lot of attention these days involves a hormone called *cholecystokinin* (pronounced kōlĭ-sĭstō-kīn′-ĭn).

Cholecystokinin is produced mainly by your intestines, and it is picked up by the bloodstream for general circulation. Its levels rise in response to the passage of fats and proteins, especially fats, from your stomach into your intestines.

Scientists have known for a long time that the hormone causes your gallbladder to contract, a fact that has nothing to do with your weight.

But recent work by Nobel Prize winner Rosalyn Yalow has stirred interest in cholecystokinin's influence on appetite. Dr. Yalow demonstrated that genetically fat rats had abnormally low levels of cholecystokinin in their brains.

Subsequent experiments involved injecting the hormone into the belly walls of both animals and humans. Immediately after the injections, the human test subjects experienced feelings of fullness and a loss of appetite, while the animals stopped eating at once.

It appears that cholecystokinin acts on the hypothalamus, and on a major nerve linking the brain and the stomach (the vagus nerve), in some way that makes you feel full. But we're still far from understanding all there is to know about this complicated hormone.

Stomach Stretching

The muscle tissue of your stomach has an elasticity that allows it to stretch temporarily as the stomach fills with food.

This stretching apparently prompts the transmission of a message of fullness from your stomach to your brain. The message evidently travels from nerve receptors in the stomach to the hypothalamus.

Your Stomach Does Not Shrink When You Diet

Contrary to a favorite dieter's myth, your stomach does not shrink when you diet. More than thirty years ago, Dr. Albert Stunkard of the University of Pennsylvania inserted balloons into the stomachs of people before and after they lost weight in order to measure the size of their stomachs. The size remained the same.

While the lining of the stomach does expand temporarily to accommodate food intake (for a maximum of about 20 ounces at one time), it neither becomes permanently larger when you overeat nor reduces in size as you start to eat less. The most likely reason for the fact that (as all dieters know) you become less hungry after a week or two of dieting is a change in hormone secretions. When external signals to get hungry are removed for a period of time, and as obesity-related hormone abnormalities that cause hunger are reduced, your "pro-hunger" hormone levels are reduced, too.

High Blood Fat

There's at least one way in which exercise may help you feel full without eating. It has to do with increasing your blood-fat levels.

There are several studies showing that high blood-fat levels are associated with feelings of fullness. The more fat you have circulating in your bloodstream, the less hungry you're likely to feel. No one is sure why.

You know that exercise stimulates the output of adrenaline and noradrenaline, and that these two hormones are powerful fat mobilizers.

By helping dislodge fat from fat cells and push it into the bloodstream, the hormones raise blood-fat levels. According to the current blood-fat theory, this makes you feel fuller.

THE EXTERNALITY THEORY

Purists might suggest a subtle distinction between "hunger" and "appetite." You could define hunger as the *need* to eat and appetite as the *desire* to eat.

This distinction figures in another approach to the question of overeating — one that has nothing to do with actual hunger or fullness. It's called the "externality theory." Simply put, the theory holds that fat people eat not so much because they're hungry, but because they like to eat.

Suppose your hypothalamus is faulty. Its signals for hunger and fullness are too low-voltage to work well. You have no accurate internal gauge to tell you when to start eating and when to stop. So you depend on external cues. If food looks good, smells good, feels good, and tastes good, you eat. You confuse real hunger with the pleasure you get from food.

External Cues

Externality theorists say that thinking about food, talking about it, and looking at pictures of it make fat people want to eat. Depression, frustration, boredom, fatigue, cold, loneliness, and discomfort make fat people want to eat. In fact, any number of emotional and physical factors unrelated to hunger seem to make fat people want to eat.

A leading proponent of this theory is Stanley Schachter of Columbia University, a respected authority on obesity. Dr. Schachter did several ingenious experiments to test his idea.

For instance, he tried shining bright lights on food to make it look more attractive. Presented with this attractively displayed food, fat people ate more than usual. Thin people were unaffected and ate their normal amount.

He set a clock ahead to indicate dinnertime. Given this external cue, fat people ate. Thin ones weren't fooled, weren't hungry, and didn't eat.

He put a group of fat people and a group of thin ones on a diet of miserable-tasting food. The thin people ate what they needed to keep up their customary calorie intake. The fat people dropped back to an incredibly skimpy average intake of 500 calories a day.

While Dr. Schachter and other experts have amassed some impressive evidence, there are other good scientists who dispute the externality theory. One of them is Judith Rodin of Yale University, another expert on obesity.

Dr. Rodin argues that most people, not just fat people, are likely to respond to tasty, attractive food. Not all fat people are overly responsive to external cues, she says, and not all thin people are immune to them. People in both groups may be highly responsive, or indifferent, or any degree in between.

Curbing the Cues

Whether entirely valid or not, the externality theory has had tremendous impact on methods for treating obesity. It has had a bearing on your life if you've had any experience with behavior modification.

Behavior modification assumes that external cues are the main cause of overeating. It reasons that you can best attack the problem by attacking the cues.

Of all the weight-control techniques aimed mainly at restricting calories, behavior modification has proved by far the most successful. For this reason, I've devoted a whole chapter to it (Chapter 14), and I heartily recommend the suggestions given there.

ALTERING YOUR APPESTAT

Curbing external eating cues should be a great help if you're trying to limit your calorie intake. But it's no substitute for strengthening your internal cues. Your first priority should be to tune up your appestat so that you'll eat when you're hungry and stop when you're full.

The only way to do this is through exercise.

You've seen how exercise fits into the various theories of hunger and fullness. But understand that the value of exercise in controlling weight is not a theory — it is a fact. The scientific evidence supporting it is quite conclusive.

Consider, for example, some experiments by nutritionist Jean Mayer, a trailblazer in obesity research. Working with overweight people, Dr. Mayer demonstrated that hard exercise depresses rather than increases appetite. He also proved that activity equaling less than the equivalent of walking three miles a day means that the hypothalamus does not operate at peak efficiency in controlling your appetite.

Once again, we see that the body seems to need a certain activity level to assure it that you're not preparing to hibernate, cross a desert, or face a famine. If you don't meet that level, your appetite increases, and the signals to stop eating become inefficient and confused.

The bottom line: *Exercise is a double-edged weapon. It causes you to burn more calories on the one hand, and to eat less on the other. This way, it satisfies both sides of the weight-loss equation.*

8.

ARE YOU FATED TO BE FAT?

"All men are created equal," our Declaration of Independence declares.

Nonsense. Obviously, we're not all equally blessed with brains, looks, social and economic advantages, educational opportunities, motivation, talent, or just plain luck. We're not created equal when it comes to fat either. In today's rabid race to be slim, not everybody has the advantage of a pole position.

Some people lag behind from the starting gun because they did a bad job of picking their parents. They inherited a potential weight problem. Others trail the field because of eating habits that date back to infancy, or even to the womb. Still others sabotage their shots at the finish line by unwittingly programming their bodies to stay fat.

FAT FAMILIES—HEREDITY OR ENVIRONMENT?

"My parents are fat. I'm doomed to be fat." So goes a common lament of fat people, and it's not without some truth.

There's no question that fat runs in families. Only 7 percent of the children of normal-weight parents grow up to be fat. But if one of your parents is fat, you have a 40 percent chance of being fat yourself. If both parents are fat, the odds go up to a really depressing 80 percent.

But as usual, statistics are better at odds than answers. What's at work here, heredity or environment? Are fat families passing on bad genes or merely bad eating habits and activity patterns? If your parents are fat, are you fated to be fat, or merely more likely to be?

Scientists have pondered this thorny problem for years. Experiments with laboratory animals have demonstrated beyond doubt that there's a genetic component to obesity. Fat mice consistently give birth to fat mice, skinny mice to skinny mice. But these findings can be applied to humans only by inference. People are not mice, and no good researcher suggests that what's true for one species must necessarily be true for a very different one.

Clearly, you can't breed people by weight categories to see if their offspring will turn out plump or puny. So scientists have taken indirect routes in search of answers. They've studied twins to see if different environments change the weight patterns of people with identical genetic legacies. They've also studied adopted children. The aim was to see if the children resembled their biologic parents or their adoptive ones in terms of weight.

The results have often been contradictory and confusing, proving mainly that people aren't nearly as predictable as mice. The debate goes on, but some conclusions are fairly clear.

When it comes to obesity, heredity versus environment isn't an either/or proposition. The two interact, and both have a bearing on whether you'll be fat.

But if you have to choose which is more important, environment is the winner. In other words, you may inherit a tendency to be fat, but that genetic destiny doesn't have to be fulfilled. Its importance is outweighed by the habits you learn from your environment.

A fat heritage may make it harder for you to be slim, but it never makes it impossible. The ultimate outcome is still up to you. Even those genetically fat laboratory mice have turned into svelte little rodents through forced alterations in their eating and exercise habits.

FROM EMBRYO TO ADULT

You can get fat at any age, and no time is ever a good time. But if you have to be fat sometime in life, choose to be a fat infant. This will give you the best chance to control your weight as an adult.

Whether an infant is fat or thin appears to have little or no bearing on whether he or she becomes a fat adult. But of children who are fat between the ages of nine and twelve, 75 percent will be fat when they're grown. And among fat adolescents, 90 percent will be fat for life.

Baby Fat

It's perfectly possible to be born fat from overeating. This has been demonstrated in children born of diabetic mothers who had abnormally high blood-sugar levels during their pregnancies. The excess sugar translated into an oversupply of food to their babies, and most of the infants were born fat.

Once into the wide world, babies establish distinctive eating patterns with amazing speed — so fast that environment can't possibly be held accountable. In one study sweetened milk was given to babies one to three days old. Some of the infants were born of overweight parents, others of normal-weight parents. Both groups seemed to like the sugared milk, and both drank it. But the babies of fat parents drank more. Crib gourmands like these may be showing traits that foretell a fat future.

Baby Feeding

One way to give a baby a slim start in life is to breast-feed it. A mother's milk flows in response to the baby's sucking. It's a sort of supply-and-demand arrangement. The mother produces what's needed and no more. The baby controls intake, drinking what it needs and no more.

The control mechanism isn't as accurate for bottle-fed babies. The baby, presented with a full bottle of milk and urged by a parent to drink it, may do just that, taking in more calories than needed.

Research has established that infants are often overfed. One problem is that parents aren't too accurate in assessing infant distress signals. A baby may cry because it's wet, restless, warm, cold, or lonely. But the usual parental response is to assume it's hungry and rush to feed it.

Parents may overfeed from selfish motives. Jean Mayer has stated that fat babies sleep more and cry less than thin ones. The slender ones are far more active, more demanding and noisier. In search of peace and quiet, parents may overload babies with food in an effort to pacify them.

Growing Up

Babies may be born with certain taste preferences. But environment soon takes an upper hand in shaping dietary habits. The substance, style, and psychology of that environment can go far to determine whether a bouncing baby will end up as a bulging adult.

Families whose diets are starchy or fat-laden, or merely overabundant, teach their children to be fat. They instill in them a taste for fattening food. Parents also teach lessons in the way they eat. If they eat big meals instead of numerous light ones, or if they gobble down high-speed meals, the child is more likely to get fat.

Parents can create potential trouble when they tangle up food with emotions, particularly with love or guilt. Using food as a reward or special treat for children is a typical bad practice. Using food to soothe hurt feelings and diminish problems is another. Parents who do this are teaching their children to associate food with love and security. This fosters an attitude that can lead to lifelong overeating. Depression, loneliness, boredom, and other forms of emotional deprivation prompt some people to stuff themselves. Psychiatrists speculate that such people turn to food for comfort because of its pleasurable childhood associations.

Also, there are adult overeaters who learned in childhood to associate uneaten food with feelings of guilt. Some of you may be familiar with the admonition: "Clean your plate. Think of the starving children in China who aren't lucky enough to have the food you do." The implicit message is that the child who leaves some food behind is somehow responsible for the fact that other children are starving. Whether this warped approach is aimed at improving the child's diet or his social conscience, it is ill advised. The ironic result may be an adult who, unable to bear the sight of a leftover, asserts his humanity by treating himself like a garbage disposal.

Finally, children are set firmly on the road to permanent fatness if they aren't encouraged by precept and example to be physically active. Sedentary children are fat children, and they become sedentary, fat adults. Children who develop an early liking for physical exertion and an enjoyment of sports have an edge toward becoming healthier, and slimmer, adults.

Twenty Percent of America's Teenagers Are Too Fat

In America, about 10 million teenagers are overweight. This comes to about one youngster in five, or 20 percent of the teenage population. Since adolescent obesity is a great predictor of adult weight problems, these youngsters are on their way to becoming the next generation of overweight Americans.

Patterns and Predictions

Childhood eating and exercise habits are likely to be permanent. If those habits are bad, fat is likely to be final. It takes an extremely strong and highly motivated person to overturn and restructure the habits of a lifetime.

The patterns that children form early are reinforced every day. They become progressively stronger over the years. The longer the patterns persist, the less subject they are to change. This is a major reason that the odds for being permanently fat increase so much from infancy through the teen years.

And breaking deeply rooted habits isn't the only problem early obesity creates. Once you've become fat, whatever your age, you've set yourself up to stay fat.

THE FAT-CELL THEORY

The reason that getting fat even once is such a handicap has to do with your fat cells. You'll remember that fat cells are where calories get stored as fat if you eat more than you need for energy and body growth and maintenance.

In 1967, Jules Hirsch, a brilliant researcher at Rockefeller University in New York, introduced a formulation that has come to be known as "the fat-cell theory." It holds that there are two different kinds of obesity. In one type, you have too many fat cells. In the other, you have a normal number, but the cells are stuffed full of fat. Scientists call the first type *hyperplastic obesity* and the second type *hypertrophic obesity*.

If you have hypertrophic obesity — overstuffed cells — your chances of reaching and maintaining a normal weight are pretty good, according to Dr. Hirsch. By reducing, you can deplete the overfilled cells and shrink them to the point of invisibility. But if you have hyperplastic obesity — too many cells — the outlook is less optimistic. Chances are that you'll lose weight with great difficulty and gain it back with great ease.

Normal Peak Periods For Fat-Cell Growth

Dr. Hirsch demonstrated that the number of fat cells increases most during the times when your body is growing fastest: in the last few weeks

Hyperplastic vs. Hypertrophic

A recent study in Sweden points up the problems of hyperplastic obesity. In the study, hyperplastic and hypertrophic obese people were put on a 20-week reducing diet. Both lost weight. But the people with too many fat cells gained weight back more rapidly than the other group. The subjects whose only problem was over-stuffed fat cells kept the weight off longer.

In a related study, the same two groups were put on an exercise program and allowed to eat as much as they pleased. The hypertrophic group lost body fat. The hyperplastic subjects didn't.

before you're born, in the first two years after birth, and in the last two years before puberty. For women, pregnancy is an additional time of rapid cell growth.

This doesn't mean that fat cells necessarily become excessive and make you fat during their peak growth periods. Rather, they increase in number to accommodate the body's changing needs.

The prenatal increase helps prepare a baby for life outside the womb. Before birth, the fetus relies on its mother's body for warmth and sustenance, so it needs no fat supply of its own. But at birth, it must be ready to fend for itself to some degree in terms of warmth and energy stores. It does this by building up a fat layer shortly before it is born.

Fat-cell increases in early childhood help supply fuel for a period of very rapid growth. And prepuberty increases aid in the body's natural transformation from the fragility of childhood into the sturdiness of adulthood. During pregnancy, increased fat cells help a woman meet the demands of supporting the growing life inside her.

Fat-cell growth during pregnancy can make for a subsequent weight problem, as you'll see in the next chapter. But this is not necessarily true of the other peak cell-growth periods. As long as you don't take in more calories than your body needs, fat cells increase only in accord with the body's growth needs, and you don't get fat.

Excessive Fat Cells

While fat-cell numbers increase most during normal growth spurts, they can also increase anytime you gain weight. It seems to work this way:

Insulin is supposed to drive fat and sugar out of your bloodstream and into your cells, as you know. The fat goes into fat cells for storage.

But if all the fat cells are full, they refuse to take any more contributions. Once this happens, you grow increasingly insensitive to insulin, even while your pancreas pours out greater and greater amounts of it. The result is that blood levels of sugar and insulin climb steadily higher and higher.

The body copes with this unhealthy situation by creating new fat cells. We don't yet know how the new cells are formed, only that high glucose and blood insulin levels seem to prompt their production.

Another mystery has to do with how fat you have to be before new fat cells are manufactured. Heredity and individual body chemistry seem to be factors here.

One theory holds that some people are born with more fat cells than others, inheriting the trait along with the color of their hair and the shape of their noses. If this proves to be true, it will go far toward explaining the genetic factor in obesity. In addition, there are researchers who believe that some people develop new fat cells more easily and rapidly than others, although there is no evidence that this tendency is inherited.

It also appears that individuals vary in how much fat they can deposit in existing fat cells before their bodies make new ones. People "lucky" enough to have overstuffed cells — the hypertrophically obese — are better off in this regard. They needn't worry about eliminating fat cells, only about emptying the ones they have.

Fat-Cell Permanence

The truly bad news in the fat-cell theory is that every new cell you form is a lifetime companion. While fat-cell numbers can always increase, it seems that they never decrease. Of course, you can empty the cells by losing weight. But you're not destroying the enemy. You're only holding it at bay. Once in place, every fat cell makes a biologic demand to stay filled.

Here I must introduce an enzyme called *lipoprotein lipase,* or LPL. Like the hormone insulin, LPL encourages fat in your bloodstream to go into your fat cells for storage. LPL is produced by empty or incompletely filled fat cells. So the more fat cells you have, the more LPL is on hand to help keep you fat.

You may have noticed that even if you have a weight problem, there seems to be an upper limit at which you stabilize and gain no more. You may also have noticed, to your sorrow, that dieting can bring on a re-bound weight gain that leaves you worse off than you were when you started.

Full fat cells produce virtually no LPL. So when your weight reaches its usual peak, there is very little LPL encouraging you to store more fat. The absence of this pro-fat enzyme helps your weight stabilize, though at a level that's probably unsatisfactory to you.

When you diet, your fat cells begin to empty. As they do, they begin manufacturing more LPL. The enzyme reaches high levels, encouraging the body to store fat rather than burn it. With the LPL scrambling to recoup lost ground, you will have to fight hard to avoid regaining weight. If you start to consume more calories than you need each day just to maintain your weight, the LPL will help see to it that those calories are stored as fat. Demoralizing as it is, this is just one more example of your body's tendency to hold its own, and then some, once you get fat.

HOW FINAL IS FAT?

Sad to report, the fat-cell theory is now less a theory than a fact. Since Dr. Hirsch first published his findings, work by others has tended to confirm their accuracy.

"The size and number of fat cells are obviously significant," concludes Dr. George Bray. "The important thing is not to let yourself get fat in the first place."

If such sage advice comes too late to do you any good, remember this: a fat-cell handicap is like the handicap of fat parents or a fat childhood. All will certainly make it harder for you to be slim. You'll cope with that fact best by facing it head-on and realizing that you'll need extra effort to overcome it.

But none of the drawbacks spells ultimate doom. If you want to be thin badly enough, and if you're willing to abandon the easy answers and deal with a hard problem realistically, no drawback will stop you.

Are you fated to be fat? Fat is persistent, insidious, complicated, and hard to handle.

But is it fate?

No. Never.

9.

THE FATTER SEX

How many of you women have heard this from a smug husband or man friend:

"I don't see why you can't lose weight. When I put on a few pounds, I can take them off in no time. It's no big deal."

The next time he says it, feel free to leave him, or threaten him with mayhem. Or offer to trade hormones with him and see if it's still "no big deal." Or show him this book. At least he'll know what you're up against.

The fact is, females are naturally fatter than males. They mature fatter, they live fatter, and they die fatter. Not heavier — fatter. Men, with their larger muscles and bones, are usually bigger and heavier. But when it comes to how much weight is made up of fat, women are easily the fatter sex.

THE GENDER BIAS

Take an average American man and an average American woman, both trim and in good shape. The man's weight will consist of 15 percent body fat, while fat will make up 25 percent of the woman's weight. In other words, if all else is equal in terms of conditioning, a woman is normally still 10 percent fatter than a man.

This is not some kind of biologic bigotry for its own sake. Women have extra fat because of their hormones. But the fact that it's natural makes it no less frustrating for a woman fighting fat. She often must work desperately hard for the same weight-control results that seem to come easily to men.

If you're a woman, you can have as many as five strikes against you before you even go to bat against fat. All but one of them involve your ability to reproduce.

Strike One: Puberty

The mere fact of becoming a woman is costly in terms of fat.

On the whole, there's not much difference in body-fat ratios between the two sexes in childhood. But when puberty starts, the scales start to tip.

A girl usually has to have about 20 percent of her weight as body fat before she can start to menstruate. This is nature's way of assuring that no baby will be conceived unless the mother has the fat she needs to carry and nourish it.

Low body fat may be why little girls who are heavy exercisers often experience "delayed menarche," or a late start in the onset of their menstrual periods. Budding ballerinas, gymnasts, and other young athletes frequently start menstruating one and a half to two and a half years later than their more sedentary peers. Their high activity level may keep their body fat too low to allow menstruation to begin.

Strike Two: Menstruation

As you know, both men and women produce sex hormones that make them characteristically male or female. For women, the two main hormones are estrogen and progesterone. Both can help make you fat.

THE MENSTRUAL CYCLE

If you're a woman, the interacting rise and fall of estrogen and progesterone are what produce your menstrual cycle. The whole cycle usually takes from twenty-five to thirty-two days. Twenty-eight days is ideal. It works like this: Your pituitary gland, located at the base of your brain, starts the ball rolling by sending out two hormones called *follicle-stimulating hormone* (FSH) and *luteinizing hormone* (LH). They cause your ovaries, your two female reproductive glands, to start producing estrogen and to ripen an egg each month.

The estrogen level is low as the cycle begins and rises steadily, peaking at about twelve days after the first day of menstruation. At this point, the estrogen stimulates your pituitary gland to release a large amount of LH, which causes one of your ovaries to release a ripe egg.

The part of the ovary that contains the egg is a bubblelike cyst called a follicle. After the follicle bursts to release the egg, what remains of the follicle is called a *corpus luteum*. This structure produces both estrogen and progesterone, which ripen the inner lining of your uterus and prepare it to nourish a potential baby.

Meanwhile, the egg, just released, is traveling through one of your Fallopian tubes toward your uterus. The Fallopian tubes are the two structures that reach from each side of your uterus in the middle toward your ovaries, one on each side of your pelvis. When the egg reaches the inside of your uterus, one of two things happens.

If the egg has been fertilized in the tube by a male sperm, swimming in the opposite direction, the egg embeds itself in the beefed-up uterine lining, and you're pregnant. Then the fertilized egg begins making a hormone called *human chorionic gonadotropin* (HCG), which keeps alive the corpus luteum in your ovary. The corpus luteum will keep making estrogen and progesterone until the placenta, or afterbirth, is capable of taking over this job. This will happen within about seven to ten weeks after your last menstrual period.

If the egg hasn't been fertilized, it disintegrates, and the corpus luteum in your ovary dies. This lets your body know that the show's over for that particular month. The estrogen and progesterone levels both drop. The uterus sheds its lining, and you menstruate. A menstrual period usually lasts for three to five days. Afterward, the cycle begins all over again.

The Hormones

Estrogen accounts for why you look like a woman instead of a man. It causes you to deposit fat in typically feminine places—the breasts, hips, buttocks, and thighs. It does this by chemically stimulating fat cells in those areas to produce unusually high amounts of LPL. You'll remember from the last chapter that LPL is an enzyme that acts like a pro-fat hormone, helping to move fat out of the bloodstream and into fat cells for storage. So the parts of the body with the highest levels of LPL are also the areas that will be fattest.

Progesterone is another female hormone. As we've discussed, its levels vary during a normal menstrual cycle, being low in the first half and high in the second half. During pregnancy, women have very high levels of estrogen and progesterone, both of which promote fatness. The main roles of progesterone are to protect the inner lining of the uterus from

Here is a graph showing how estrogen and progesterone rise and fall at various phases of the menstrual cycle:

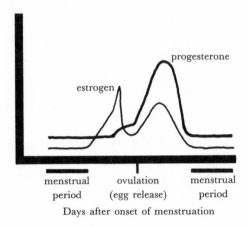

getting overstimulated by the hormone estrogen and to prepare the inner lining of the uterus for a pregnancy. But progesterone affects your appetite and mood too.

Progesterone is a *catabolic* hormone. This means that it tends to break down protein. It also makes you hungrier, although scientists don't know why. Many women tend to eat more in the second half of the menstrual cycle, and many develop ravenous appetites during pregnancy. Mothers-to-be often eat far more than they need for themselves and their babies, and this excess food makes them fatter. Progesterone or some of its by-products makes you feel sluggish and sleepy, less inclined to exercise.

Unlike progesterone, the primary male hormone, testosterone, is *anabolic*. This means that it promotes muscle growth. Men normally have high levels of testosterone, while women normally have very low levels of this hormone. So men have a natural tendency to become lean and muscular, while women have a natural tendency to become fat.

The more muscle you have, the larger your appetite is likely to be. As you know, your body's yellow-fat tissue is mostly dead weight. It requires and consumes very few calories. On the other hand, lean tissue — the type that makes up your muscles and organs — consumes a great many calories to keep you alive and functioning. Since a well-functioning hypothalamus tries to keep calorie intake balanced with body needs, it mandates a big appetite for people with a lot of lean tissue. This is why most men, who are more muscular, normally eat and expend more calories than most women, who are fatter.

In addition, both estrogen and some by-products of progesterone cause you to retain fluid. They act on the kidneys to help them keep salt in your body, and salt causes water to be held, too. This can make your rings and shoes feel tight during the few days just before your period begins. It's common for women to feel uncomfortable at this time of the month. Fortunately, the water retention and other discomforts are temporary. When estrogen and progesterone levels fall, leading to menstruation, the excess water is eliminated through urination, and the other uncomfortable sensations disappear too.

Strike Three: Contraception

If you're a woman practicing birth control, you may be taking the Pill. Despite a growing public wariness about possible side effects, birth-control pills are still the most popular form of contraception in America.

The Pill is fattening.

There are different types of pills, but the one most women use is called the "combination" pill. It's a combination of synthetic estrogen

---

Birth-Control Pills

• LOW ESTROGEN

Brevicon
Loestrin 1.5/30
Lo/Ovral
Modicon
Ortho-Novum 1/35

• VERY LOW ESTROGEN

Loestrin 1/20

• NO ESTROGEN

Micronor
Nor-Q.D.
Ovrette

---

and progesterone. You take it for twenty-one days, then stop for a week to have your period. This pill prevents pregnancy by making your ovaries less likely to release an egg and by making it difficult for sperm to reach any egg that is released.

There are lots of brands of pills. They differ mainly in their concentrations of estrogen and progesterone. A pill may have more of one and less of the other, or more of both, or less of both.

The Pill is fattening for the same reasons your body's own, natural estrogen and progesterone are. Fortunately, the most popular pills used today contain much less estrogen and progesterone than the older pills, which were the only ones available until recently. The newer ones are much less fattening and much safer, too.

Strike Four: Pregnancy

This is the big one. If the Pill can make you pudgy, pregnancy can make you elephantine.

To begin with, you have to gain a certain amount of weight if you're to have a successful pregnancy. A woman who's at normal weight before conception should gain at least 20 pounds to nourish her baby properly. Anywhere between 20 and 35 pounds is about right for most pregnant women. The total includes extra fat, along with the weight of the baby, the fluid it rests in, and the placenta that feeds it.

But if you're overweight before pregnancy, you still should gain weight. Gaining less than 20 pounds during pregnancy increases your chances of giving birth to an abnormal or small baby.

So make sure that you reduce *before* you become pregnant. Pregnancy is no time to try to lose weight.

PREGNANCY AND HORMONES

Whether you need to gain weight during pregnancy or not, the odds are that you will. You'll get plenty of encouragement from your hormones. Your progesterone levels stay high from the beginning of your pregnancy to the end. So instead of making you hungrier for a few days each month, the progesterone stimulates your appetite without letup for nine months.

A second hormonal problem has to do with insulin. You'll remember from Chapters 4 and 6 how weight gain tends to make you resistant to insulin. This also happens during pregnancy. Your fat cells become more and more insensitive to insulin. So your pancreas produces it in ever-increasing amounts in order to clear your blood of excess sugar and fat. Your insulin levels are higher, and more of the food you eat is converted and stored as fat.

The insulin problem repeats itself with every pregnancy. The more children you have, the more times you're exposed to this fat-adding process, and the more fat you may gain.

PREGNANCY AND FAT CELLS

But neither progesterone nor insulin is the worst villain when it comes to weight gain during pregnancy. That distinction belongs to fat cells.

As you know, both sexes add fat cells during certain periods of rapid growth. And both men and women can add them anytime they gain weight rapidly. But with pregnancy, women have a high-risk period for fat-cell increase that men never have to contend with.

It's the extra fat that usually comes with pregnancy, not the pregnancy itself, that increases your number of fat cells. How many you add depends on how much and how fast you gain fat. The number of pregnancies doesn't appear to matter. If you gain more fat with your first pregnancy than your fifth, your first will be more costly in terms of added fat cells.

Of course, most women do gain extra fat in pregnancy. But each added fat cell is there for life, always demanding to be filled. This is the main reason some of the weight gained in pregnancy tends to hang on so tenaciously long after the baby is born.

Nevertheless, if you are pregnant and already overweight by more than 20 to 35 pounds, you should *not* attempt to start a reducing diet. Trying to lose weight during pregnancy can result in the production of ketones that can cause brain damage in the fetus. Weight loss also can cause stunted fetal growth and other abnormalities.

Strike Five: Inactivity

When you were a little girl, did your parents encourage you to play with dolls, or climb trees? Were you praised for being pretty, or for running faster than any other kid on the block? The point is this: as a woman, you live in a culture bent on keeping you simpering and sedentary.

Of course, things are changing. Lately, women are gaining more of their rightful respect as athletes, and more women are taking pride in keeping their bodies fit. But for most of our history, only males were encouraged to be physically active — strong, fast, venturesome, and skilled in sports. For women, physical achievement was viewed as being somehow unfeminine.

One result of this attitude was generations of out-of-shape American women. Society added a cultural burden to the physiological ones nature had already built in. This made women even more fat-prone than they naturally are.

The welcome change in cultural attitudes toward women and exercise is solving part of the inactivity problem, but the dilemma is building on another front. Technology has seen to that.

The last few decades have seen a staggering increase in the number of gadgets designed to lighten the workload traditionally allotted to women. Consider: dishwashers, clothes washers, dryers, vacuum cleaners, electric can openers, floor polishers, and on and on. The list is virtually endless.

While the gadgets may make women happier, they also tend to make them fatter. Labor saved means calories unspent. And stored calories mean stored fat.

SPECIAL HEALTH PROBLEMS OF OVERWEIGHT WOMEN

Fat presents some health problems that are for women only.

Cancer

You saw in Chapter 4 how obesity can make a woman more likely to contract uterine cancer, and breast cancer as well.

Fat tissue has the ability to convert a woman's androgens (male-type hormones) to estrogens, and many overweight women with irregular menstrual periods have high estrogen levels and low progesterone levels. Estrogen stimulates cell growth and makes cells even more responsive to estrogen. Progesterone counteracts estrogen by preventing cell overgrowth and making cells less responsive to estrogen. Too much estrogen and too little progesterone can lead to excessive cell growth, which constitutes cancer.

Abnormal Menstruation

A fat-related overabundance of estrogen can also disrupt your menstrual cycle, either partially or completely. When obesity prevents the release of an egg, estrogen is produced, but progesterone is not. Progesterone is needed to properly ripen the inner lining of your uterus and prepare it for menstruation. Lack of progesterone prevents proper ripening and the menstrual period that follows.

Infertility

There may be another factor in an overweight woman's failure to menstruate, and this one can limit or eliminate her ability to conceive.

Obesity can interfere with the monthly release of an egg by several mechanisms that are not completely understood. This can happen either occasionally, or every month, depending on the individual. Obviously, you can't get pregnant in any month when no egg is released.

I can't tell you exactly how fat you have to be for your menstrual cycle and your fertility to suffer. Some women are regular and fertile at 300 pounds, while others stop menstruating and become infertile at 150 pounds. In any case, any problem with menstruation or fertility should prompt you to see your gynecologist.

Difficult Pregnancy

The most common problems associated with pregnancy in obese women are diabetes and high blood pressure, both of which I described in Chapter 4. These can be dangerous to both mother and child.

Obese women also are more likely to develop gallstones, blood clots, and varicose veins. In addition, few are able to avoid the extra discomfort that excess fat inflicts on them during pregnancy.

Pregnancy alters almost every woman's spinal alignment to some degree. Your protruding belly pulls your spine forward, bending your back out of its usual shape. Obviously, obesity may exaggerate this condition. With extra weight beyond that of the fetus tugging on your spine, you're likely to develop persistent backaches.

You may have frequent and severe leg aches and joint pains as well, as your body protests the added load of pregnancy on top of the excess weight it already carries. And you'll be more awkward and tire more quickly than a thin pregnant woman.

Difficulty in Childbirth

Too much maternal fat can complicate delivery for mother and baby alike.

Your doctor may have difficulty starting intravenous feeding or medication for you because your veins are obscured by a thick layer of fat. The injection of spinal anesthetic may be unduly hard, again because excess fat hinders the needle from reaching its target.

The complications of obesity in pregnancy can lead to difficulty in childbirth, too. Diabetes, for instance, can be hard to control during labor and delivery. This means that your blood sugar will fluctuate widely, rising too high and falling too low. Your newborn may become sick as a result of these fluctuations. Poorly controlled diabetes throughout pregnancy can cause your baby to become large, so large that its head or shoulders may not fit easily in your birth canal. Your baby may be injured during the birth process, and you may need a cesarian section to avoid such injury.

Obese women are usually out of shape and because of this get short of breath and tired before the baby is born. Labor and delivery are hard work. You have to contract your muscles actively and bear down to push the baby through the birth canal. This may be too much work for you if you're out of shape.

If you need stitches, for either a vaginal delivery or a cesarian section, obesity will prolong your healing time.

If your obesity causes high blood pressure, and frequently it does, you may need medication to control your blood pressure. And that can affect your baby.

GOOD NEWS AT LAST

Now that you've heard all the gloom and doom about women and fat, Lord knows, ladies, you need a lift.

Here it is: it's just possible that the fat women among you are more sensual — more sexually responsive — than your skinny sisters.

I say "possible" because there's no conclusive scientific proof. The only study I know of on the subject took place a few years ago at Michael Reese Hospital in Chicago. Researchers there looked into the reported sexual responses of two groups of thirty women each. One group consisted of fat women, the other of slender ones.

Women in both groups reported about the same frequency of sexual activity. They made love about nine times a month. But while the thin women usually said they were satisfied with their sex lives, the fat women were not. A statistically huge majority of the fatter women said they wanted more sex than they got.

The study found that in terms of sexual excitability, the fat women outscored the thin ones almost two to one. The investigators concluded that the fat women "obviously weren't overeating instead of having sex; their craving for both food and sex exists almost simultaneously."

If fat women are really more sensual, the reasons are anybody's guess. The Chicago researchers speculated that fat women may have more psychological hunger in general. In other words, they may want more in the way of food, sex, love, comfort, warmth, or just about any other kind of pleasure you can name. This may be because of some personality pattern in fat people that science has yet to establish.

Or there could be some physiological connection between being fat and being sensual. It's possible that the part of the brain that controls the appetite for food controls other appetites as well. If this is true, then a woman who enjoys food a great deal will also enjoy sex a great deal.

Or the explanation may lie with some kind of evolutionary holdover from the days of the fat and flirtatious cavewoman.

In any case, where do men fit into all this? If fat women are sexpots, are fat men more sensual as well? Probably not, but they may not be any less so, either. Although obese men have lower levels of testosterone and higher levels of estrogen than do thin men, the fat ones appear to have normal sex drives and potency.

10.

POUNDS AND PREJUDICE

WITH some 40 percent of Americans over their ideal weights, we're right to be concerned, even alarmed, about obesity. But there's another pathology at work today that should alarm us as well. This growing, spreading, social malady includes such victims as:

- A college coed from a wealthy family who, convinced that she is "too fat," starves herself to death.
- A young woman suffering from a host of illnesses who finally confesses to her doctor that for five years she has been taking forty laxatives a day, every day, to "control her weight."
- A man with an IQ in the genius range who is denied a job with a large corporation because of his weight. His girth puts him at odds with the corporate image of a lean go-getter.

These are not isolated cases. Together, they represent the experiences of hundreds of thousands of Americans who have fallen prey to our extreme prejudice against fat.

THE NEW BIGOTRY

"It is no longer fashionable to look down on people because of the color of their skin or the length of their names or the shape of their noses," says obesity expert Jean Mayer. "It is unfortunately very fashionable, however, to look down on the obese as weak-willed individuals. The prejudice is very strong, and is expressed in every possible way."

Dr. Mayer did a survey on how fat people are viewed by academia, which presumably represents the more enlightened among us. He found that fat girls have only one third the chance of being accepted into top-rated American colleges as slim ones. Only two obese boys get into the best colleges for every three normal-weight boys with similar grades and credentials.

Another obesity authority took note of our extreme bias in a paper published in the *Annual Review of Medicine* in 1981. Faith T. Fitzgerald of the University Hospital at the University of Michigan put it this way:

"It is clear from reading magazines or watching television that public derision and condemnation of fat people is one of the few remaining sanctioned social prejudices in this nation freely allowed against any group based solely on appearance.

"It has been documented that all of us — the general public, social workers, employers, graduate schools admissions officers, nurses, and physicians — feel negatively toward the obese," Dr. Fitzgerald continued. "Obesity is a moral crime and one of the few remaining sinful diseases: One is fat because of 'weakness of the will.' The fat are denied jobs, promotions, educational opportunities, and, recently, challenged in their right to adopt a child until they lose weight."

And from researcher Jack Kamerman of the Department of Sociology and Social Work at Kean College of New Jersey: "Fat people are expected to participate in their own degradation by agreeing with others who taunt them. If any other stigmatized group were similarly derided on television and radio or in movies, lawsuits would result."

Fat and Social Class

Our prejudice against fat people contains an element of classism. We associate sleek leanness, especially in women, with wealth, opulent tastes, exclusive fashions, and jet-set lifestyles. Obesity, on the other hand, is equated with shabbiness, squalor, and poverty.

These equations are not without some basis in fact, for scientists have discovered an enormous correlation between fat and social class in America. They have found that by and large, obesity is a problem of the poor and underprivileged — at least among women.

Studies show that the weight of men tends to rise with favored social and economic status. In other words, a middle-class man is likely to be fatter than a poor one, and a rich man will be still another rung up in terms of heftiness.

On the other hand, quite the reverse is true for women, who make up the majority of our obese population. Among women the richer you are, the more entrenched you are socially, the less likely you are to be fat.

Landmark work in this area was done by Dr. Albert J. Stunkard of the University of Pennsylvania, a renowned researcher on obesity. He and his associates did a research project in New York called the "Midtown Manhattan Study." Among other things, the study found that a lower-class woman was six times more likely to be fat than an upper-class woman. Thirty percent of the women in the survey's lower socioeconomic group were obese, 16 percent of those in the middle class, and only 5 percent of those in the upper class.

The study also showed that obesity in women was rarest among Protestants with ancestry of long tenure in America. Thinnest of all were white Episcopalians, a group traditionally associated with elite social status. Among Jewish women, Catholic women, immigrants, and daughters of immigrants, obesity was commonplace. (The study did not cover blacks or American Indians, but other surveys have found these two groups to be among the fattest of all Americans.)

The Midtown Manhattan findings were so consistent and so statistically significant that Dr. Stunkard formed a startling conclusion: second only to heredity, socioeconomic status is the single strongest determinant of whether a person will be fat or thin. This may be because class standing has something to say about how hard a woman will try to conform to the social ideal of slenderness.

Fat and Morality

Snobbery may explain some of our prejudice against the obese, but not all. It can scarcely account for the vehemence of the scorn that many feel for fat people or the irrational strength of the antifat prejudice.

People who would never think of discriminating against someone on the basis of color, religion, ethnic origin, or sex nevertheless treat fat people with profound contempt. The reasoning seems to be that while no one can escape a condition of birth such as sex or ethnic heritage, being fat is "a matter of choice." Presumably, people are fat because they "lack the gumption" to do something about their weight. They are "willfully" affronting society with their excess pounds.

But *what* social taboos are fat people breaking to earn themselves such a stigma? Surely they must be treading on something more sacred than mere aesthetic taste.

BODY VS. SOUL

You may already have spotted a clue to a possible answer in Dr. Fitzgerald's perceptive remark that "obesity is a moral crime and one of the few remaining sinful diseases."

Most of us grew up with the idea that there is something bad, something wrong, about the flesh and its hungers. This view is, of course, a very old notion in our culture — as old, in fact, as Judeo-Christian thought, if not older. Specifically, the Puritan world-view that forms the ethical bedrock of American culture holds that each of us is a battlefield for two warring factions. On one side is the body. On the other is the "soul," or "spirit," or "mind." The spiritual side is "pure," while the body — the fleshly or carnal side — is "evil," "sinful," "corrupt." In the old Puritan view, the body had to be scourged, chastened, and subjugated lest its appetites endanger the salvation of the soul.

Maybe it's only a coincidence that the thinnest Americans are also those with the longest, deepest, and closest ties to our culture's Puritan heritage — to the ethic that preaches self-denial. But it's hard to keep from suspecting that the notion that fat people are "weak-willed" is really a mask for the old Puritan worry that the flesh is a lot stronger than the spirit would like it to be. In fact, if flesh is bad, having too much of it must be morally significant — it implies that the obese have succumbed to their carnal natures! They are gluttonous, weak-willed, self-indulgent. They are fat because they take a lot more pleasure than they should in food. They are fat because they sin.

A NEW TWIST ON THE OLD MORALITY

Millions of Americans are still zealously trying to subdue the flesh, in a very literal way — by getting rid of it. Slenderness and fitness are the watchwords of the new religion. Physical perfection is the new salvation. And we pursue it with all the Puritan fervor and evangelical style that once fueled the sermons of our hellfire-and-brimstone Puritan forebears.

Diet messiahs abound. Each propounds the virtues of his or her system with the passion of a tent preacher seeking converts. Each promises life-altering results from weight loss. Each has his or her own band of faithful disciples spreading the quick-loss gospel to the heathen, exhorting them to repent of their fatness and forsake their high-calorie ways.

Being thin is not only beautiful. It is righteous.

Fat and Pop Psychology

The fat-sin equation owes at least some of its durability to modern pop psychology. The present-day popular version of the old doctrine holds that the sinners — fat people who overeat and underexercise — are fat because they're "depressed" or "anxious" or somehow mentally unhinged; for "sin," we now substitute words like "neurosis," or "emotional instability," or "social maladjustment." This is just the old Puritan bugbear back in a new guise — for the underlying implication, once again, is that fat people wouldn't *be* fat unless they were inwardly deficient in some way.

The casting about for psychological demons to exorcise has led to mountains of research to pin down some link between mental or emotional problems and obesity. But results have failed to bear out the popular assumption.

Research has shown that from a mental-health standpoint, the obese are pretty much like everyone else — no crazier, no more neurotic, no more anxious or depressed, no less stable, and no more "maladjusted." They're not especially "jolly," as the old stereotype would have it, nor are they by nature especially unhappy.

It is true that many fat people associate food with gratifying childhood emotions — love, security, comfort. So do many thin people. It is also true that many overweight people report that they eat when they're depressed, anxious, bored, or frustrated. Some even say that eating is the only activity that relieves their anxiety about their weight. But thin people may also respond to emotional stress by overeating. The difference is not in the stress reaction itself. It lies, rather, in the degree and frequency of stress-eating episodes and in the ability to handle them emotionally and metabolically.

BODY IMAGE DISTURBANCE

While fat people aren't necessarily unhappy by nature, this is not to say that they're happy about being fat. Being fat may very well make them unhappy for the perfectly sound reason that society punishes them unreasonably for their weight problem. Being the object of social contempt for any reason is hardly likely to make someone happy.

Dr. Stunkard, a psychiatrist himself, has found that persons in good mental health are unlikely to suffer any great emotional trauma from being fat. Fat-related mental problems seem to arise when other, nonrelated, emotional factors are at work. For instance, people who feel rejected by their parents might focus their anger and frustration on the fact that they're fat. They conclude that their weight is what makes them unlovable.

For some people fat may even become the symbol and focus of all their problems. They see themselves as enormous, elephantine, grotesque. The severe form of this distorted self-image is known technically as "body image disturbance." People who suffer from it blame all their troubles and failings on their size. They often believe their lives would change magically if they could only get down to some arbitrary ideal weight.

Most victims of this distorted self-concept are people who were fat adolescents. Thoughtless cruelty from parents and peers can be devastating at that particularly vulnerable time. Even well-meant efforts to "help" fat teenagers by urging them to reduce, or telling them how attractive they could be if they lost weight, can be as clumsy and damaging as outright malice. "You have such a pretty face" can leave just as deep a scar as "You look like a pig." Both imply that a person is not acceptable as he or she is.

And the scars are slow to heal, particularly for women. Studies show that the few fat adolescent girls who manage to reduce and stay thin as adults are not emotional success stories. They spend their lives in constant anxiety about their weight. They diet constantly. They become terribly upset at gaining only two or three pounds. Many are unduly preoccupied with how they look. They may continue to see themselves as fat long after they've achieved and sustained an ideal weight.

PREJUDICE AND FAT WOMEN

Women are not only the fatter sex. They are also the sex that worries more about being fat and suffers more from the prejudice against fat people.

Studies show that an extra 15 or 20 pounds cause a woman to worry about her weight, while a man gets concerned only when his excess fat amounts to 35 pounds above the national average. Women make up between 90 and 95 percent of the membership of diet organizations in America. Of the 5,000 people each year who have their intestines shortened to lose weight (see Chapter 18), 80 percent are women. *Anorexia nervosa* and *bulimarexia* are dangerous patterns of weight-related obsessive behavior that I'll discuss later in the chapter. Their victims are, almost exclusively, women.

The New Feminine "Ideal"

The special vulnerability of women to the social prejudice against fat is the subject of a poetic and insightful book by California author Kim Chernin. It is called *The Obsession: Reflections on the Tyranny of Slenderness.*

In it, Ms. Chernin — who appears to share my view about the Puritan element in our antifat prejudice — takes on one of the strangest paradoxes of our time: why is the age of women's liberation also the age of a desperate obsession to minimize the female body? At a time when women are seeking to enlarge their opportunities and expand their horizons, they are trying even harder to diminish and reduce their very flesh, "to turn away from whatever is powerful in women." The mere hint of the rounded hips or prominent breasts that once inspired worship now makes a woman horrified at being "fat."

Ms. Chernin theorizes that as women have begun to assert themselves, they have increased the threat they pose to men. A large woman, she says, is a threatening woman to those who unconsciously fear the more assertive feminine ideal that has been evolving with the growth of the women's movement. As we learned in previous chapters, almost every society throughout history has viewed the rounded, well-fleshed feminine body — that is, the female in her mature, postadolescent form — as womanly and desirable. But now, Ms. Chernin reasons, this version of feminine beauty is becoming an unconscious threat to many people. Result: this woman is being replaced by the skinny, immature, and therefore nonthreatening, child-woman — the woman who looks less like a woman and more like an adolescent boy.

The author makes a good case for her theory. She notes, for instance, that:

- Fashions have become increasingly geared to the adolescent and preadolescent figure. Today's most popular models are often prepubescent girls. Boyish figures dominate advertising in magazines and on television.
- Movies such as *Pretty Baby* and *Taxi Driver*, whose sexy heroines are child prostitutes, are both popular and critically applauded.
- Child pornography is enjoying an unprecedented vogue. Incest and child

molesting have emerged from the closet to become hot media topics and vehicles for popular literature.

"In this age of feminist assertion men are drawn to women of childish body and mind," Ms. Chernin concludes, "because there is something less disturbing about the vulnerability and helplessness of a small child — and something truly disturbing about the body and mind of a mature woman."

It is even sadder to note that women are willing accomplices to their own defeminization. They accept the imperative of extreme thinness as natural and right.

Anorexia

If slenderness is our new cult, victims of anorexia nervosa are its pathetic fanatics. Anorexia (from the Greek word for absence of appetite) is a mental disease characterized by willful self-starvation. Unless successfully treated, it is usually fatal.

Anorexics are almost always female. They are often from middle- or upper-middle-class families. They are usually adolescents or young women, achievement-oriented perfectionists — model students and model children.

Contrary to their name, anorexics are not without appetite. They live with a desperate hunger. But their sole, obsessive joy lies in mastering that hunger in the name of conformity to the ideal of slenderness. Ironically, anorexics usually see themselves as "too fat" even while they emaciate themselves, even when they no longer carry enough fat to sustain life.

Anorexia was once very rare. Today it is considered by many experts to be epidemic.

Bulimarexia

Like anorexia, bulimarexia is a new medical phenomenon, so new that the name for the disease was only coined in the 1970s. *Bulimarexia* is more or less synonymous with *bulemia* (from the Greek words for ox and appetite), although bulemia originally referred only to compulsive overeating or binge eating.

Now both terms are used to describe a "binge-purge" syndrome. Bulimarexics — again, almost always women — gorge themselves with food, then get rid of it with self-induced vomiting or with laxatives, or with both. One of the milder symptoms of the compulsive vomiter is rotting teeth. Digestive juices erode the tooth enamel.

Severe bulimarexia can be fatal. Drastic and frequent purging can cause mineral imbalances that can lead to irregular heartbeats and death.

Many anorexics are also bulimarexics. Like anorexia, bulimarexia has become a common disease. And like anorexia, it is a disease whose causes are as much sociological as psychological.

CAN PREJUDICE HELP KEEP YOU FAT?

The answer is yes. The real irony about our antifat bias is that it probably does as much to perpetuate obesity as it does to eliminate it.

Losing weight is a very hard thing to do. To be successful at it in a healthy and lasting way, a robust optimism and a good self-image are almost essential. Unfortunately, many fat people lack these weapons because they accept society's illogical judgment — that they're fat because they have some moral or psychological flaw.

Of course, this is not the case. Like all prejudices, the antifat bias reflects ignorance. In truth, obesity is a problem with complex and often mysterious causes, causes that have little if anything to do with psychological quirks, weak will, or moral turpitude.

If you're fat and miserable about it, let guilt be the first weight you drop. Recognize the antifat prejudice for what it is: misguided and destructive. Then turn your liabilities into assets.

Instead of being ashamed of your body, be proud of your courage in confronting and fighting a difficult problem with sane eating and exercise. If you fall off your weight-loss program from time to time, don't undermine yourself with silly recriminations. Lapses can and do happen to everybody. Just take up where you left off.

If your failure to conform to society's standard of slimness bothers you, fine. Use your vanity as another spur to help you toward your goal. There's nothing wrong with wanting to look your best. If you're a woman, you needn't accept the dictum that looking good means looking like an undernourished adolescent boy. The mature female body is beautiful and miraculous.

Finally, never lose sight of the true issue: *your health.* Enjoying your body fully and preserving it longer require that you reach and maintain a satisfactory weight.

Don't do it just because society says you must. Do it for yourself. You're worth it.

11.

CALORIES AND NUTRIENTS: WHAT YOUR BODY NEEDS

How many of you have tried to lose weight on a high-protein diet that was very low in carbohydrates? If you stayed on it long enough, you probably found yourself so weak that you could hardly walk across a room. So you quit the diet, and you gained weight.

What about a high-carbohydrate diet that was very low in protein? Eventually, you may have found your hair falling out, your skin scaling, and your fingernails splitting and chipping. So you quit the diet, and you gained weight.

There's an important lesson in such an experience: *your body needs a variety of foods — a balanced diet — to stay healthy. A diet that is out of balance is self-defeating. It will not make you permanently slender, and it may very well make you sick.*

Any diet that restricts calories, including an unbalanced diet, will probably make you lose weight in the short run. But if you stay on a lopsided diet long enough, you'll be forced to choose between the diet and your health. If you're wise, you'll abandon the diet rather than risk illness. For most people, this means returning to old, fattening eating habits. The inevitable outcome is a disheartening and dangerous regain of weight.

Obviously, then, the only sane and effective weight-loss diet is a balanced diet — a diet you can follow for a lifetime to regulate your weight without risking your health.

I've outlined such a diet for you in Chapter 13. But don't rush ahead to it. You'll have more success with the diet if it makes sense to you — if you understand the logic behind it. Take time with this chapter to learn some of the basics of good nutrition. Get to know what foods you need, how you use them, and how you can best spend a low-calorie allowance.

WHAT IS A BALANCED DIET?

A balanced diet is one containing all the food components your body needs to maintain itself and run properly. These components are called *nutrients*. The criterion for deciding what constitutes a nutrient is this: will the absence of the substance in question endanger your health?

Experts using this guideline have determined that the adult human body requires forty-six nutrients. If you lack any one of them, sooner or later your health will suffer.

Water is a nutrient, and it constitutes a nutrient category all by itself. The other forty-five nutrients are divided among five more categories — carbohydrates, protein, fat, vitamins, and minerals. Three of these groups — carbohydrates, protein, and fat — contain calories.

I can see you dieters wincing at the very mention of the word. Calories, the enemy! You should readjust your thinking. Even when you're trying to lose weight, you need a certain number of calories. They're the fuel your body runs on, and they go hand in hand with many vital nutrients.

Success in dieting doesn't just mean limiting calories; it means limiting calories without sacrificing nutrients.

The 46 Essential Nutrients

- Water
- Glucose
- Linoleic acid
- 9 amino acids
- 13 vitamins
- 21 minerals

CALORIES

Although calories are supplied by three of the six nutrient groups, calories are not nutrients in themselves. Calories are energy. A calorie is the energy in food, expressed in terms of heat. As we commonly use the word, a *calorie* is the amount of heat needed to raise the temperature of one liter of water by one degree centigrade.

Energy needs vary enormously among individuals. However, let's say that the average active, normal-weight American man takes in about 2,800 calories a day. His female counterpart consumes about 2,100 calories a day. These average people maintain stable weights because they work off enough calories each day to avoid accumulating any surplus energy to be stored as fat.

But suppose you want to reduce your weight, not merely maintain it?

To do this, *you must run up a calorie deficit: you must burn more calories than you take in.* This is the all-important equation in the arithmetic of weight loss. You must eat less, and at the same time you must exercise more. Exercise burns more calories while you do it and long after you have stopped.

Remember, you must do both. You've already seen how dieting without exercise only sets you up for the perilous yo-yo syndrome of quick loss and quick gain.

But how drastically must you curtail your calories?

For most people, the daily food intake should never drop below 1,300 calories. This is the minimum you need if you're to exercise effectively, and it's the minimum that allows you to get all the nutrients you need.

Are All Calories Equal?

You will store extra calories as body fat, no matter where those calories come from. You may get them from carbohydrates, protein, or fat, or any combination of the three. Your body has the ability to convert *any* foodstuff to fat, just as long as the energy in that food totals more energy than your body needs.

But this is not to say that the source of your calories doesn't matter at all. In deciding how to spend an allotment of 1,300 calories a day, keep two facts in mind:

- Carbohydrates in the form of vegetables, fruits, and whole grains are the least fattening type of food you can eat. High-protein foods tend to be somewhat more fattening. Fat is without doubt the most fattening food of all.
- Fortunately, the same food order that guides you in restricting calories guides you in balancing your diet. For good nutrition, you need more carbohydrates than protein, and you need fat least of all.

Relative Calorie Values

Fat has 9 calories per gram, while carbohydrates and protein each contain about 4.5 calories per gram. On the face of it, it seems clear that carbohydrates and protein are about equally fattening, and each is only half as fattening as fat.

But for several reasons, these measurements don't tell the whole story.

One reason lies in the calorie "packaging" of different types of foods. Are calories tightly packed in a small volume of a certain food? Or does the food give you a lot of volume at a low cost in calories?

Fat is not only intrinsically high in calories, but is also a source of *densely packed* calories. A mere tablespoon of butter, a high-fat food, has 100 calories. For the same cost in calories, you could eat two heads of lettuce. The choice is between a mere condiment, however tasty, and a whole meal of a filling vegetable.

Except in their purest form, which is sugar, carbohydrates give you a lot more volume per calorie than other foods, so you can eat more of them without getting fat. This is especially true of vegetables and fruits. They get much of their bulk from water, which has no calories. They also gain bulk from fiber, a nonfattening kind of carbohydrate you'll learn about later in the chapter.

Generally, high-protein food is a much denser source of calories than carbohydrates, though less so than fat. Consider steak, which many people wrongly regard as a good "diet" food. In fact, a small, lean steak has upwards of 400 calories. For the same price in calories, you could eat a huge vegetable salad with three tablespoons of oil and vinegar dressing.

Your Body: A Calorie-Burning Processing Plant

There's another factor that helps clarify the picture of the relative calorie values of carbohydrates, protein, and fat. This has to do with the energy your body must expend to process a particular food; that is, to change it from its original form into stored body fat.

To understand this better, compare your body to a refining plant, perhaps a plant that turns crude oil into heating oil. If the plant gets high-grade crude, it can turn out the finished product with only a few, relatively inexpensive processing steps. But if the raw material is low-grade crude, more processing is required, at a cost of more labor and expense.

In these terms, fat is the highest-grade raw material for the body, followed by carbohydrates and then protein.

It's so easy to turn fat in your food into stored body fat that only 6 percent of the calories in the fat you consume in food is used up in the process.

Carbohydrates require a little more work. So they lose on the order of 15 percent of their calories in the conversion from food to body fat.

Protein is toughest of all. Protein relinquishes 25 percent of its original calories to cover the cost of processing.

From the standpoint of processing, then, protein is the least fattening type of food, followed by carbohydrates. And fat is once again the most fattening of all.

Unknown Factors

Nutritionists generally agree that carbohydrates are the least fattening

---

FOOD AND NUTRITION BOARD, NATIONAL ACADEMY (
DAILY DIETARY ALLOWANCE

Designed for the maintenance of good nutrition of practica

	AGE (YEARS)	WEIGHT (LBS.)	HEIGHT (IN.)	PROTEIN (G)	FAT-SOLUBLE VITAMINS[a]			WATER-	
					VITA-MIN A (μG)	VITA-MIN D (μG)	VITA-MIN E (MG)	VITA-MIN C (MG)	THI MIN (MG
Males	11–14	99	62	45	1000	10	8	50	1.
	15–18	145	69	56	1000	10	10	60	1.
	19–22	154	70	56	1000	7.5	10	60	1.
	23–50	154	70	56	1000	5	10	60	1.
	51+	154	70	56	1000	5	10	60	1.
Females	11–14	101	62	46	800	10	8	50	1.
	15–18	120	64	46	800	10	8	60	1.
	19–22	120	64	44	800	7.5	8	60	1.
	23–50	120	64	44	800	5	8	60	1.
	51+	120	64	44	800	5	8	60	1.
Pregnant				+30	+200	+5	+2	+20	+0.
Lactating				+20	+400	+5	+3	+40	+0.

Adapted from Recommended Dietary Allowances, revised 1980, Food and Nutrition Board, Natio Academy of Sciences, National Research Council, Washington, DC.

food type, followed by protein and fat. But they don't know all the reasons why this is true.

It's obvious why fat is the most fattening. It has the most calories per gram, it has the most densely packed calories, and it loses the fewest calories in processing.

But the situation is murkier when it comes to carbohydrates and proteins. After all, they start off calorically equal in pure form. And while carbohydrates are less dense calorically, protein loses more calories in processing. Suppose you tried two weight-loss diets identical in calories — one high in protein and the other high in carbohydrates. Logic indicates that you'd lose slightly more weight on the high-protein diet.

But there is considerable evidence that the logic doesn't bear out in practice. Scientists have done experiments putting animals on diets that were different in content but *equal* in calories. Though they ate no more calories, the animals getting most of their calories from fat turned out to be fattest. The animals feeding mostly on protein were next highest

SCIENCES—NATIONAL RESEARCH COUNCIL RECOMMENDED REVISED 1980
all healthy people in the U.S.A.

SOLUBLE VITAMINS[a]					MINERALS[a]					
RIBO-FLAVIN (MG)	NIACIN (MG)	VITAMIN B_6 (MG)	FOLACIN (μG)	VITAMIN B_{12} (μG)	CALCIUM (MG)	PHOSPHORUS (MG)	MAGNESIUM (MG)	IRON (MG)	ZINC (MG)	IODINE (μG)
1.6	18	1.8	400	3.0	1200	1200	350	18	15	150
1.7	18	2.0	400	3.0	1200	1200	400	18	15	150
1.7	19	2.2	400	3.0	800	800	350	10	15	150
1.6	18	2.2	400	3.0	800	800	350	10	15	150
1.4	16	2.2	400	3.0	800	800	350	10	15	150
1.3	15	1.8	400	3.0	1200	1200	300	18	15	150
1.3	14	2.0	400	3.0	1200	1200	300	18	15	150
1.3	14	2.0	400	3.0	800	800	300	18	15	150
1.2	13	2.0	400	3.0	800	800	300	18	15	150
1.2	13	2.0	400	3.0	800	800	300	10	15	150
+0.3	+2	+0.6	+400	+1.0	+400	+400	+150	[b]	+5	+25
+0.5	+5	+0.5	+100	+1.0	+400	+400	+150	[b]	+10	+50

[a]Amounts in μg are in micrograms (one-millionth of a gram); amounts in mg are in milligrams (one-thousandth of a gram).
[b]Supplement of 30 to 60 milligrams generally recommended for these groups.

in weight. The animals eating mostly carbohydrates were slimmest of all.

So far, we are at a loss to explain why protein turned out to be more fattening. Whatever the reason, though, one fact is clear: of the three nutrient groups with calories, carbohydrates provide the highest bulk value for the fewest calories.

Budgeting Your Nutrition Allowance

The most important consideration if you're budgeting calories is how much nutrition you're getting for what you spend.

It's quite true that carbohydrates, protein, and fat are all necessary to a balanced diet. But you don't need them in equal proportions.

The ideal diet for nutrients would consist of about 60 percent carbohydrates, about 15 percent protein, and less than 25 percent fat. Compare this to the average American diet, which is bountiful but hardly balanced: only 40 percent carbohydrates, 16 percent protein, and a whopping 40 to 45 percent fat!

As you can see, we Americans would be better off nutritionally if we increased our carbohydrate intake, ate less protein, and curtailed fat drastically. We would also be much slimmer.

CARBOHYDRATES — THE SUGARS YOU CAN'T DO WITHOUT

Carbohydrates are food components that are made up of carbon, oxygen, and hydrogen (hence the name, carb-o-hydrate). More simply put, carbohydrates are sugars.

Carbohydrates may exist as single sugar molecules, or as two or more sugar molecules bound together. The single sugars are called *monosaccharides*. Two sugar molecules bound together are called *disaccharides*. *Polysaccharides* are found in food as chains of hundreds of thousands, or even millions, of sugar molecules joined together. Disaccharides and polysaccharides must be broken down into monosaccharides before your body can use them.

Monosaccharides (Single Sugars)

There are many single sugars in foods. But only four — glucose, fructose, galactose, and mannose — can pass from your upper intestine into your bloodstream. We'll call these four the "acceptable" sugars.

All other monosaccharides — as well as all disaccharides and all polysaccharides — must be broken down chemically in the upper intestine into one of the four acceptable monosaccharides before proceeding for further processing.

Once they leave your intestines, the four acceptable sugars head for your liver via a large blood vessel called the *portal vein*. The portal vein is the sole avenue for blood leaving the intestines, and it goes only to the liver.

Where Sugars Are Found

Glucose and fructose are found separately in fruits and honey. They are found bound together as sucrose in table sugar. Galactose is found bound to glucose as lactose, the sugar in milk. Mannose is rarely found in foods but is used in research because it can pass from the intestines into the portal vein without preliminary processing in the intestines.

Glucose may pass unchanged through the liver to circulate throughout your bloodstream. But fructose, galactose, and mannose must be picked up by your liver and changed to glucose before reentering the bloodstream.

The bottom line is this: all the carbohydrates you eat, from corn to candy bars, end up as glucose before going into general circulation for use by your body.

Disaccharides (Double Sugars)

The most important double sugars are *lactose*, which is found in milk, and *sucrose*, which is granulated table sugar.

Disaccharides are broken down in the upper intestine into single sugars before entering the portal vein. If they can't be broken down, they go to the lower intestine and are fermented by bacteria to form gas.

Sugar Circulation

All carbohydrates are sugars bound together. They can be single sugars as in fruit and honey; two sugars bound together as in milk and table sugar; and hundreds and thousands of sugars bound together, as in corn and beans.

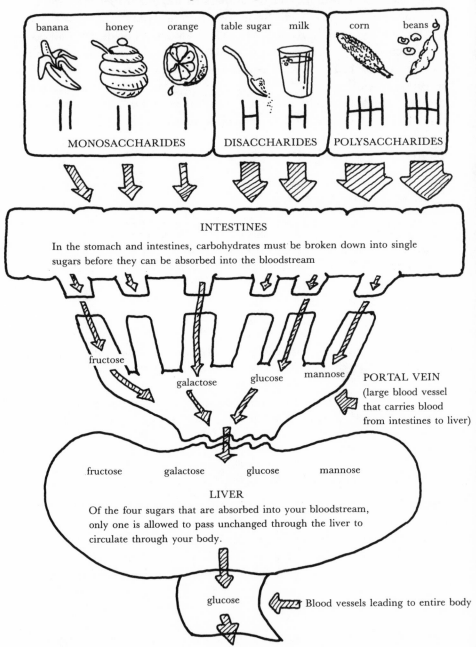

All carbohydrates eventually end up as glucose before they can circulate through your body.

Polysaccharides (Multiple Sugars)

Polysaccharides, or multiple sugars, occur in food in two forms. One is *starch*. The other is *fiber*, or *cellulose*.

STARCH

Starch consists of sugar molecules bound together in hundreds, thousands, and millions. Most starches break down easily into single sugars in your upper intestine, so they're readily absorbed for use by your body. Starch that can't be absorbed in the upper intestine goes to the lower intestine and ferments to form gas.

Starch is found in abundance in "starchy" foods such as beans, corn, potatoes, and rice.

FIBER

Fiber, or cellulose, is made up of millions of sugar molecules bound together in chains. High-fiber foods are the "complex carbohydrates" you may have read about, and they're good news for dieters.

Food has to be absorbed before its energy can be converted to body fat, and fiber is almost impervious to absorption. Your upper intestine can't break it down at all. Bacteria in the lower intestine break it down only slightly. So by and large, fiber passes out of your body in your stool little changed from the way it came in. It leaves behind very few calories.

Fiber makes up much of the bulk of fruits and leafy vegetables. This is largely why these foods offer a lot of volume for only a few calories and are therefore great for dieters. Fiber also adds bulk to your stool and thereby helps prevent constipation.

There's still another bonus to a high-fiber diet. As the fiber passes through your intestines, it picks up a certain amount of calorie-rich fat. The fat, unabsorbed, passes out of your body along with the fiber. So if you must have a pat of butter, eat it on a piece of high-fiber bread, which is bread made from whole grains. This way, you'll probably absorb fewer calories from the butter.

Why You Need Carbohydrates

Carbohydrates are your basic fuel for movement. They're the main source of energy for your muscles when you exercise. Since exercise is the key to weight control, carbohydrates are essential to any weight-loss diet.

Going on a low-carbohydrate diet to lose weight is ridiculous. You're only sabotaging yourself by curtailing your capacity to exercise.

MUSCLE FUEL

You'll remember from Chapter 3 that your body can run either on sugar or on fat. The sugar comes from the carbohydrates you eat. The fat is either fat you eat or stored body fat that you mobilize for energy. However, your body can convert sugar to fat if fat is what your energy needs dictate.

Fat's main advantage as a fuel is that the body can store vast reserves of it. Sugar's main advantage is that it's more efficient. Burning fat requires a lot of oxygen, while burning sugar requires less.

This is why your muscles burn sugar almost exclusively during all-out exercise, when oxygen is at a premium. When you're resting and oxygen is plentiful, your muscles burn almost 100 percent fat. Between extremes the fuel mix goes on a sliding scale, depending on your degree of activity or inactivity.

FUEL SOURCE VS. ENERGY EXPENDITURE

Don't be misled here. The fact that your muscles burn fat while at rest does *not* mean that you can lose body fat by lying in bed. What matters is not the type of fuel being used, but the amount of energy being expended.

Remember, weight gain or loss is governed by the balance between the energy — or calories — that you take in as food, and the energy you expend for body maintenance and movement. Regardless of the fuel being used, you burn only about 40 calories per hour when you're resting. Compare this to the 800 calories you burn in an hour's worth of hard running.

The fat you burn while resting is quickly replaced by fat in your food, or by the liver's releasing stored fat or sugar that it has converted to fat.

What Your Liver Does with Glucose

But how does glucose get to your muscles to be used as energy or to your fat storage depots to be stored as fat? Let's return for a moment to the story of how carbohydrates are processed.

When last we looked in on the liver, it was humming away to convert all incoming monosaccharides to glucose, if they weren't glucose already. What does the liver do with all that glucose? There are four choices:

- It can use the glucose to provide itself with immediate energy. After all, livers work hard.
- It can convert the glucose to fat and store it. The fat can be released later for energy or be stored elsewhere in the body as body fat.
- It can store the glucose as such, to be doled out into the bloodstream later.
- It can release the glucose into the bloodstream for immediate distribution. Cells throughout the body then pick up the glucose and burn it for fuel.

As you can see, glucose always ends up either as immediate energy or potential energy. Glucose is the only nutrient that carbohydrates provide. But its importance as an energy source can hardly be overstated.

GLYCOGEN
When glucose arrives to be stored in the muscles as potential fuel, it is called *glycogen*, or muscle sugar. The endurance of your muscles depends on how much glycogen they can store before you start to exercise.

If you're on a very low-carbohydrate diet, you won't be able to exercise very hard or very long, if at all. Your muscles will have so little glycogen to fuel them that the slightest activity will tire you.

BRAIN NOURISHMENT
In addition to fueling your muscles, carbohydrates are vital to your brain. As you learned in Chapter 3, your brain feeds almost exclusively on glucose.

Your blood carries only about three minutes' worth of glucose at any given time. But your brain needs a continual supply. So your liver works constantly to keep up with the demand. Even so, the liver itself can store only about twelve hours' worth of glucose.

This is why you must eat breakfast. After an overnight fast, your liver is short of stored glucose to parcel out for your brain. Breakfast replenishes the store. Even when you're dieting, don't deprive yourself of a high-carbohydrate breakfast. Without it, your brain may run short of glucose. If it does, you may feel tired and weak, or even dizzy and faint.

Avoiding Excess

As useful as carbohydrates are, you don't want to overdo them. Like any other foodstuff, carbohydrates in excess are converted to fat and stored as body fat.

With any type of food, the watchword is balance. Carbohydrates should make up the largest single segment of your diet, but they are not the only type of food you need. The proportions you'll find in the Getting Thin Diet, explained in the principles behind the diet, are the ones you should follow for optimum nutrition.

PROTEIN

While Americans may not eat a disproportionate amount of protein, we do seem to be oversold on the benefits of this particular type of food. When we go on diets, we often spend an unnecessarily large portion of our calories on high-protein food. After all, we've been assured by many diet gurus that this is the healthy thing to do.

Protein is certainly a valuable source of essential nutrients, but it doesn't live up to some of the extravagant claims made for it.

For instance, protein is not a magical muscle-builder, as many athletes used to believe. You strengthen your muscles through certain kinds of exercise, not through eating outsized amounts of any special foodstuff. If you take in more protein than you need, all it does is make you fatter — not firmer or more muscular.

Protein is not uniquely suited to a good weight-loss diet either, despite such claims by proponents of high-protein regimens. As you've learned, protein is a rather dense source of calories. In Chapter 13 you'll find out how to get all the protein you need at a relatively cheap cost in calories.

What Is Protein?

Protein is the basic structural material for all plant and animal bodies. It is made up of *amino acids*. Amino acids are the building blocks of all the tissue in your body. Your hair, your skin, your muscles, your internal organs are all composed in part of amino acids.

Protein contains the element nitrogen. Carbohydrates and fat don't.

For this reason, your body can't convert the carbohydrates and fat you eat into protein. However, the conversion process can go the other way. Your liver can knock off the nitrogen in protein and convert what's left to fat or sugar.

Where Essential Amino Acids Come From

Animal protein—meat, fish, poultry, eggs, and milk products—contains all nine essential amino acids. Vegetable protein is usually missing one or more. In other words, eating a single vegetable may give you fewer than nine.

But even vegetarians can get all the essential aminos by combining vegetables with other vegetables and with other products. For instance, neither corn nor beans have all nine essential amino acids. But the two in combination do.

Different cultures have learned how to get the nine essential amino acids without using animal protein. Mexicans, for example, have a tasty dish made from corn tortillas and beans, which together provide all nine essential amino acids, as does a favorite Oriental dish containing bean sprouts and rice.

Here are some other combinations that will give you all nine:

Peanuts and	Barley
	Bran
	Corn
Soybeans and	Oats
	Rice
	Rye
Beans and	Sesame
	Wheat
Leafy vegetables and	Most grains and cereals

Since it can be changed into energy-producing substances, protein can be used for energy — but only indirectly. It is never a source of immediate energy, as fat and carbohydrates are, because it requires extra processing.

Protein is made up of twenty-two amino acids, but only twenty-one of them are found in humans. Of these twenty-one, nine must come from your diet. Your body can manufacture the other twelve. Because the nine dietary amino acids can't be made internally — either at all or in adequate amounts — they're called the "essential" amino acids. You must be sure to get enough of them in the food you eat. With the Getting Thin Diet, you will.

How You Use Protein

Your body uses the building blocks of nutrient groups to supply its needs. In carbohydrates, the building blocks are sugars. In protein, they are amino acids.

Just as carbohydrates must be broken down into single sugars, protein must be broken down into single amino acids before your body can absorb and use it.

The breakdown takes place in your stomach and upper intestine, and the single amino acids go to your liver. That endlessly clever organ then decides what to do with them:

- It can recombine them to make new protein that your body needs.
- It can route the amino acids into your bloodstream to be picked up by other parts of your body and used as needed — as hair, skin, hemoglobin, muscle, or any number of other types of tissue.
- It can eliminate or convert excess amino acids. Your body has no way of storing protein, so any surplus must either be eliminated or converted to fat or sugar. If you have too much protein, the liver breaks down each amino acid into two basic components, nitrogen and organic acids. The nitrogen becomes ammonia to be eliminated by your kidneys in your urine. The organic acids may also pass out of your body via the kidneys. But if you're really overloaded with protein, your liver and kidneys won't eliminate all the organic acids. In this case, the liver converts them to sugar or fat to be used for energy or stored. Thus the converted organic acids can wind up as body fat, just as excess carbohydrates and fat you eat can.

How Much Protein Do You Need?

Since so much of your body is made up of protein, you need protein to keep your tissue vital and healthy.

But this is not to say that you absolutely must eat protein every day. Your protein tissue is in a constant state of flux, building up and breaking down. It is always giving up its amino acids and then recombining them to form new tissue. Used amino acids can be recycled, combining with one another or with new amino acids coming in from your food to build new tissue.

For example, some of the protein in muscle tissue replaces every single amino acid in its structure every four days. If your body needs some other kind of protein tissue in a hurry, it can use the amino acids being released from the muscle tissue — or any other tissue — and recombine them to form whatever new tissue is needed.

If all the amino acids in your body could be kept there and recycled indefinitely, you'd never need protein in your diet. But of course, this is not the case. Some amino acids are always being lost. This is why you can't go for very long without protein in your diet.

If you become deficient in protein, your hair will begin to fall out. Your skin will be rough and scaly. Your nails will be fragile and grow very slowly. Your lips will dry and peel.

But these are minor problems compared with the dangers posed by a severe and protracted protein deficiency. In this case, your various body tissues, scavanging for what little protein is available, feed off one another. As your lean tissue gives up its protein and fails to replace it, it weakens. Your muscles shrink. Your organs, including your heart, begin to fail. Eventually, you die.

Fortunately, death from protein deficiency is very rare in America, where high-protein food is abundant.

Adequate protein need not be expensive or hard to get. The body can get by quite well with only the daily protein ration found in two large glasses of milk, or in 12 ounces of corn and beans. You don't have to eat meat, fish, chicken, or eggs. Virtually everything you eat has some protein, since protein is in every single cell of every plant and every animal.

Though Americans don't usually go to extremes in their protein consumption, we're more likely to eat too much than too little. And eating too much creates problems of its own.

Since you can't store protein, your liver and kidneys have to work overtime to process it and get rid of the excess. Remember, protein is the hardest foodstuff for your body to process. A diet markedly overabundant in protein causes the liver and kidneys to enlarge. If your liver and kidneys are normal, this probably won't hurt you. But if either is diseased, you can get very sick and perhaps even die.

And, once again, you can get fat. Protein has calories — often quite a lot of calories. And calories from any source can end up as body fat.

FAT

As you know, fat is far and away the most fattening of the calorie-bearing nutrient groups. It is, alas, also the best tasting to most people. Experiments on animals and humans have shown that mammals overwhelmingly prefer the taste of fatty foods to any other taste.

We Americans are crazy about fat. We cook our food in it, and we often embellish food with it. Butter, mayonnaise, gravies, sauces, salad dressings, sour cream — all those things that turn plain food into very tasty food are rich in fat and loaded with calories.

We are by no means unique in our love for fat. Natives of virtually every culture that has easy access to fat eat it in abundance. Perhaps the human taste for fat is another holdover from the days when storing body fat was a great advantage. In her zeal to preserve the species, nature may have given us a taste for the most fattening food possible.

The Fat Cost of Fast Food

Fast food may taste good and save you time and money, but from a dieter's standpoint the price is high. Here's how some popular fast-food meals break down in the ratio of fat to total number of calories consumed:

	CALORIES	% OF CALORIES FROM FAT
Burger King Whopper, fries, and vanilla shake	1,250	43
McDonald's Big Mac, fries, chocolate shake	1,100	41
Arthur Treacher's fish and chips (2 pieces fried fish, fries, cola)	900	42
Arby's roast-beef plate (roast-beef sandwich, 2 potato patties, coleslaw, chocolate shake)	1,200	30
Pizza Hut 10-inch pizza with three toppings	1,035	35
Kentucky Fried Chicken (3 pieces chicken, potato, gravy, coleslaw, roll)	830	50

Compiled by author from information supplied by companies.

The American diet is far too rich in fat. We would do well to cut our fat intake by at least half. But even dieters shouldn't avoid fat altogether. You need it for the energy it provides, for its essential tissue-building properties, and for the way it helps you use other nutrients.

What Is Dietary Fat?

The fat you've been reading about throughout most of this book is stored body fat, the kind you may be trying to shed. Keep in mind that the fat I'm discussing now is *fat in your diet*, a different thing altogether.

Dietary fat is defined as chemicals that can't be dissolved in water. Fat has many constituents, including fatty acids. These are the only building blocks of fat that need concern us. There are scores of different fatty acids. They can be stored or burned for energy, or they can be converted by your body's cells to cholesterol and triglycerides, the blood fats you learned about in Chapter 4.

Dietary fat can be subdivided into visible and invisible fat. The visible fat is the kind you see in meats and other greasy foods. Oil is also a visible fat. Invisible fats are less obvious in appearance and texture. They are found in nuts, pastries, avocados, and many processed foods.

How You Process Fat

Fat is broken down in your intestines into elemental particles composed mostly of fatty acids. These can pass directly from your intestines into your bloodstream, but not without some help. Since fats can't dissolve in the water that makes up most of your blood, they sneak in under camouflage. Proteins in your intestines combine with them and form protective shells around them. Encapsulated in this way, the fats enter your bloodstream and circulate throughout your body. The fats bound to proteins are called *lipoproteins.*

Once in your bloodstream, fats can go into any cell in your body to be burned for energy or used as part of the cell itself, or they can go into fat cells for storage.

But remember, it's not only fat from fatty food that ends up in your fat cells. Your liver can make fat from either protein or carbohydrates. The issue once again is how much total energy you're accumulating — not the source of that energy. You need fat in your diet, just as you need protein and carbohydrates.

Why You Need Fat

Linoleic Acid
There are many different fatty acids that your body uses. It can manufacture all but one by itself. The one you need to get from your food is called *linoleic acid*.

Linoleic acid is a building block for the manufacture of cell membranes for all the trillions of cells in your body. It is also a building block for sex hormones. In addition, linoleic acid is vital for proper hormone functioning.

Fat's Other Uses
As you know, fat is the main fuel for your muscles when you're inactive or sleeping. But you really don't need dietary fat as an energy source. Your body can get all the fat energy it needs by mobilizing your stored body fat and burning it.

However, dietary fat is needed to maintain a certain level of fat in your intestines. Without intestinal fat, you couldn't absorb certain vitamins at all, and some minerals would be difficult to absorb.

Vitamins D, E, and K, and some of vitamin A, are fat-soluble. This means they can dissolve only in fat. They must be dissolved in order to enter your bloodstream. If you had no fat in your diet, you could become deficient in the fat-soluble vitamins, and possibly in some minerals as well.

Finally, you need dietary fat for the healthy functioning of your immune system. You'll recall that your immune system protects you from invading organisms, from virus and bacteria to carcinogens. Recent studies show that people on very low-fat diets may be more susceptible than other people to immune defects and certain types of cancer.

How Much Fat Do You Need?

If you eat the typical American diet, you're eating a lot more fat than you need. In fact, you could probably cut out all visible fats and still never become fat-deficient. You would get enough dietary fat from grains, nuts, and other vegetable matter.

There are considerable risks in a diet that's too high in fat.

It can, for instance, increase your chances of developing cancer of the colon, or large intestine. The more fat you take in, the more bile your liver produces. Bile, a breakdown product of fat metabolism, is secreted by the liver into the intestines. An overabundance of bile is associated with cancer of the colon.

A high-fat diet may also be linked to cardiovascular diseases. Scientists used to think that such a diet might be directly responsible for heart attacks and other cardiovascular problems. This may not be exactly the case. It may be that the fat poses a hazard only when it's part of a diet that is also too high in calories. The incidence of heart attacks is very low in some societies whose diets are high in fat but low in calories.

But a diet high in both fat and calories — a diet common in America — is dangerous. It can cause hardening of the arteries, strokes, heart attacks, and kidney failure.

Even nondieters should, therefore, try to limit their fat intake. You might try eliminating, or reducing, the ice cream, butter, margarine, and whole milk in your diet. Go easy on mayonnaise and fatty salad dressings. Learn how to broil and boil food as alternatives to frying it. Don't eat the skin of any animal, fish, or fowl, since skins are loaded with fat.

The Saturated Fat–Cholesterol Controversy

Like many people, you may be concerned about your intake of *saturated fats* (fats that become firm at room temperature, and are found in whole milk products, animal fats, and certain oils) and *exogenous cholesterol* (that is, cholesterol that comes from the foods you eat, as opposed to HDL and LDL, the two types discussed in Chapter 4, which are manufactured by the body).

Exogenous cholesterol is found in high amounts in eggs, liver, hard cheese, red meats, and all animal fats. It can add to the amount of LDL ("bad") cholesterol in the blood. For this reason, scientists have thought that lowering the amount of exogenous cholesterol in the diet might lower the risk of heart disease and other illnesses associated with LDL.

Recently, scientists have come to believe that saturated fats are more to blame than exogenous cholesterol for raising the level of blood cholesterol. For some years, health experts recommended that *unsaturated fats* (fats that stay liquid at room temperature, which means most vegetable fats and oils) be substituted for saturated fats.

The opinion of many nutritionists and health experts now, however, is that by far the most important thing you can do for your health is to cut back your intake of *all* fats — saturated, monounsaturated, and polyunsaturated — from the American average of 45 percent to a more reasonable (though perhaps still not ideal) intake of less than 30 percent.

VITAMINS

Of course, anyone on a diet should eat less. But to be healthy, you must get all your essential nutrients from the foods that you eat. Although you should eat fewer carbohydrates, and less fat and protein — which all contain calories — you must eat enough to assure a proper supply of vitamins and minerals. Along with water, vitamins and minerals make up the three noncaloric nutrient groups.

What Are Vitamins?

Essentially, most vitamins are chemicals that combine with other chemicals to form *enzymes*. Enzymes are *catalysts*. A catalyst is a substance that has to be present for a particular chemical reaction to take place. Without a catalyst, the reaction would take place slowly, or not at all.

As components of enzymes, vitamins help you process other nutrients, and they facilitate a wide range of other vital chemical reactions in your body.

For example, three B vitamins have to be present for your body to break down sugar for energy. Without them, you couldn't metabolize the sugar properly. And your brain, which gets more than 98 percent of its energy from sugar, would be in danger of starvation.

Vitamins are present in most of the food you eat. They pass directly from your intestines into your bloodstream after they've been dissolved, either in water or in fat.

How Many Vitamins Do You Need?

Americans are wildly overenthusiastic about vitamins.

A catalyst provides the environment necessary for a certain chemical reaction to occur. But, though it must be present, the catalyst doesn't *cause* the reaction. Since it's not a direct participant, hardly any of the

Vitamins

Thirteen vitamins are essential in the human diet. This chart lists each vitamin, what it does, deficiency symptoms, and the food sources for each one.

VITAMIN	WHAT IT DOES	DEFICIENCY SYMPTOMS	FOOD SOURCES
A (retinol)	Helps maintain skin, eyes, urinary tract, lining of the nervous, respiratory, and digestive systems. Needed for healthy bones and teeth.	Scaling of skin; small bumps around hair follicles, eye irritation, impaired night vision, possible eventual loss of vision; frequent colds and coughs; sometimes loss of senses of taste, smell. Kidney stones.	Sweet potatoes, milk, liver, fish liver, oils, eggs, butter, green and yellow vegetables.
B₁ (thiamine)	Needed for carbohydrate metabolism and release of energy from food. Helps heart and nervous system function properly.	Impaired nerve function—tingling, pain, loss of feeling; possible loss of muscle control; possible shortness of breath, rapid heartbeat, heart failure. Psychologically, possible diminished reasoning capacity, depression, loss of memory.	Yeast, meat, whole-grain and enriched breads and cereals, nuts, peas, potatoes, most vegetables, citrus fruits.
B₂ (riboflavin)	Helps body cells use oxygen. Promotes tissue repair and healthy skin.	Sore throat, cracking of skin of lips; redness and rawness of tongue, scaly rash on body; anemia and abnormal nerve function with pain, tingling, numbness; cataracts, causing possible loss of vision. Psychologically, possible sense of dislocation.	Milk, cheese, liver, fish, poultry, green and yellow vegetables.

(continued)

VITAMIN	WHAT IT DOES	DEFICIENCY SYMPTOMS	FOOD SOURCES
B₃ (niacin)	Essential for cell metabolism and absorption of carbohydrates. Helps maintain healthy skin.	Pellagra—a disease characterized by scaly red rash that may spread over body; mouth ulcers, severe diarrhea; headache, dizziness; insomnia, depression; loss of muscle control; loss of sensation; unexplained pain due to nerve impairment.	Liver, yeast, lean meat, whole-grain and enriched breads and cereals.
B₆ (pyridoxine)	Needed for healthy teeth and gums, blood vessels, nervous system, red blood cells.	Scaly rash on face and scalp; redness, pain in tongue; swelling of joints with pain, tingling, numbness. Psychologically, sense of dislocation. Later, may include anemia, seizures.	Yeast, whole-grain cereals, meat, poultry, fish, most vegetables, citrus fruits.
Pantothenic acid	Helps body convert carbohydrates, fats, and proteins into energy.	Headache, fatigue, insomnia, nausea, abdominal cramps, vomiting, gas; loss of muscle control; pain or loss of sensation due to nerve impairment; muscle cramps; burning sensation in feet.	Egg yolk, meat, nuts, whole-grain cereals.
B₁₂	Essential for proper development of red blood cells. Helps in proper function of nervous system.	Anemia; nerve degeneration with pain, loss of sensation, loss of muscle control; shiny tongue; possible irreversible damage to central nervous system.	Eggs, meat, milk, milk products.

Biotin	Needed for healthy circulatory system and for maintaining healthy skin.	Same symptoms as for pantothenic-acid deficiency, above.	Egg yolk, nuts, liver, kidney, most fresh vegetables; is made by intestinal bacteria.
Folacin (folic acid)	Needed for production of red blood cells.	Anemia; nerve degeneration with pain, loss of sensation, loss of muscle control.	Green leafy vegetables, citrus fruits, yeast, meat, poultry, fish.
C (ascorbic acid)	Essential for sound bones and teeth. Needed for tissue metabolism and wound healing.	Early: red bumps around hair follicles; later, scurvy: bleeding from gums, nose, or elsewhere, teeth that loosen, may fall out; eventual anemia and death.	Citrus fruits, tomatoes, raw cabbage, potatoes, strawberries, cantaloupe.
D (calciferol)	Essential for calcium and phosphorus metabolism.	Gradual softening of bones, with gradual bending of leg bones; bones likely to fracture under very little stress.	Fish-liver oils, fortified milk, eggs, tuna, salmon, sunlight.
E (tocopherol)	Helps prevent oxidation of polyunsaturated fatty acids in cell membranes and other body structures.	Rupturing of red blood cells and weakening of muscles. Vitamin E deficiency is very rare.	Whole-grain cereals, lettuce, vegetable oils.
K	Needed for normal blood clotting.	Excessive bleeding due to inability of blood to clot; nosebleeds; exaggerated bruising.	Leafy vegetables; is made by intestinal bacteria.

Columns 1, 2, 4: Victor Herbert, M.D., from Nutrition Cultism (Philadelphia: George F. Stickley Co., 4th printing, 1980), pp. 174–175. Reprinted by permission. Column 3: Dr. Gabe Mirkin.

catalyst gets used up in the reaction. So most of the catalyst's components, including vitamins, are available for recycling.

This is why most people don't need vitamin supplements. Vitamins last a long time in the body, and those that are depleted are easy to replace. The National Academy of Sciences has established a recommended daily allowance, or RDA, for each vitamin. The RDAs for most vitamins are readily available in the standard American diet.

Anything extra is a waste. You need only so much and no more of a vitamin to facilitate any given chemical reaction. Having more than you need won't make the reaction take place any better or any faster. The excess will simply present your body with another disposal chore. For example, when you take a large dose of vitamin C, some 80 percent of what you absorb ends up in your urine shortly after you take it.

But if you think your diet may be deficient in one or more vitamins, and you want to cover all the bases, go ahead and take a daily multiple vitamin pill. The dosages in such pills aren't high enough to cause any trouble. At worst you'll only be wasting money and excreting vitamin-rich urine.

Beware, however, of exceeding the RDAs appreciably. An overabundance of some vitamins can be dangerous, or even fatal.

For instance, too much vitamin A can cause joint pain and bone breakdown. Massive doses of vitamin C can trigger kidney stones and cause kidney damage. Too much vitamin D can cause the calcification of your arteries and muscles. Too much vitamin B_3, or niacin, can cause liver damage and ulcers. Vitamin E overdoses can cause liver damage, high blood pressure, and blood clots.

MINERALS

What Are Minerals?

Minerals are basic chemicals found in the soil and in the air. They're taken in by growing plants. Animals get them by eating the plants, or by eating animals that eat the plants, or both. Humans usually get them by eating both.

Twenty-five minerals are essential to human life. Four — carbon, hydrogen, oxygen, and nitrogen — are structural components of the food

The Minerals Essential for Life

Carbon	Oxygen
Hydrogen	Nitrogen

MAJOR MINERALS	TRACE MINERALS	
Calcium	Fluorine	Nickel
Phosphorus	Silicon	Copper
Chlorine	Vanadium	Zinc
Potassium	Chromium	Selenium
Sulfur	Manganese	Molybdenum
Sodium	Iron	Tin
Magnesium	Cobalt	Iodine

you eat. Therefore, they are counted separately in calculating the number of essential nutrients.

The twenty-one essential minerals we *do* count are not structural parts of your food, although you take them in along with your food. Seven of these are needed in large amounts in your diet. The other fourteen are needed in much smaller amounts and are called *trace minerals.*

Minerals enter your bloodstream by diffusion through your intestinal walls.

Why You Need Minerals

Minerals are necessary to everything that goes on in your body because they enable electrical conduction to take place.

Remember our discussion of the human electrical system in Chapter 6? Every bodily activity runs on electricity, and minerals supply the battery. Just as in a battery, activity in the body occurs when an electrical current passes from an area of greater mineral concentration to an area of lesser concentration.

In addition to enabling conduction, minerals help you store water, and they determine how the water is to be distributed in your body. They help control your body's heat buildup. And finally, minerals, like vitamins, are building blocks for the enzymes that enable vital chemical reactions to take place.

Essential as they are, minerals in overabundance can be perilous. For example, overdoses of potassium can stop your heartbeat. Too much iron can severely damage your liver, heart, and pancreas.

Do You Need To Take Extra Minerals?

The only mineral supplements that I recommend for healthy people are iron for women during their childbearing years and calcium after menopause.

Men get all the iron they need through their diets. Women would too if they didn't menstruate. But the extra iron lost through menstruation makes one out of every four women in this country iron-deficient even if she is not anemic. If you feel tired or rundown, it may be a good idea to ask your doctor for a blood test to measure the amount of iron in your bloodstream and the levels of the proteins that carry iron in your blood. If you are iron-deficient, you should take extra iron.

Some postmenopausal women, growing less active with age, may curtail their food intake to avoid the weight gain that can come with a more sedentary lifestyle. All women are at risk of incurring a calcium deficiency, a condition that helps account for a high incidence of bone softening in women over fifty.

It may take as long as fifteen years for a gradual loss of calcium to become serious. But by the time it does, your bones may be so soft that they break easily.

The condition can be avoided by maintaining good nutrition as you age. But if you feel your diet may be lacking in calcium, ask your doctor to test you to see if you're losing more calcium than you should. If the doctor recommends a calcium supplement, follow that advice.

SALT

Salt is not a mineral in itself. Rather, it is a combination of two minerals, sodium and chlorine. It deserves separate mention in our discussion of minerals because of the increasing concern among doctors about the overabundance of salt in the American diet.

You need only about 200 milligrams of salt each day. But most Americans take in between 6,000 and 18,000 milligrams a day — thirty to ninety times what they need. Even if you stopped salting your food, cooking with salt, and eating anything with a salty taste, you would still take in about 3,000 milligrams a day. This is more than enough for anyone, even for regular exercisers, who lose large amounts of salt through their sweat.

We Americans take in large portions of salt in part because of our dependence on processed, canned, and frozen foods. Manufacturers of these products routinely add salt, either as a preservative or as a flavoring agent. For example, canned peas contain more than 300 times as much salt as fresh ones.

The problem with our salty diet is that it can lead to high blood pressure. Salt helps the body retain water, and a higher level of water in the body means a higher blood volume coursing through veins and arteries. About one American in five develops high blood pressure, which is a risk factor in heart attacks, strokes, and hardening of the arteries.

Unfortunately, the damage done to many people who eat too much salt it not readily reversed. For reasons as yet undiscovered, reducing salt intake will not return a high blood pressure to normal in most cases. As you can see, then, it's a good idea to cut back on your salt intake as much as possible before problems have a chance to develop.

WATER

You already know what water is and why you need it. Water is a compound of hydrogen and oxygen, and you need it to live. Water is the most essential nutrient of all.

It's possible to live for about sixty days without food and all the nutrients and calories food provides. But five days is the absolute upper limit that any human being can survive without water. On a hot day, with no water available, you can die of dehydration in less than twenty-four hours.

Water normally makes up 65 percent of your body weight. It is a component of every one of your cells. It makes up most of your bloodstream. It is the basic medium that carries all the other nutrients throughout your body. Nothing functions without it.

How Much Water Do You Need?

You're always losing water from your body, and you must keep replacing it. Thirst is normally a pretty good regulator of how much fluid you drink, so most people get the right amount to replace what they lose.

Every day you lose a little more than five pints of water, and every day you take in roughly the same amount.

You lose almost three pints of water in your urine. Almost two more pints are lost from water vapor breathed out of your lungs and evaporated off your skin, even when you're not sweating. You lose about one fifth of a pint a day in your stool.

You must be especially careful to replenish water on a day when you're sweating heavily. Sweating can cost you another one to twenty pints of water in a day.

You replenish about three pints of water a day from drinking it and drinking other liquids. Another two pints or so come from eating the many foods that contain water. A tomato, for example, is about 80 percent water. Another one-half pint is produced by your body daily as a by-product of metabolism.

BEWARE OF FADS

Now that you understand more about the relationship between your body and its food, you should be armed to resist the more outrageous fad diets. You know now that a diet that preaches deficiency — or excess — in any nutrient is potentially dangerous and ultimately useless.

If you still have any doubts about that, read the next chapter.

12.

PROBLEM DIETS: HOW NOT TO EAT

"My long-range goal is to get the Nobel Prize for having discovered the cure for fat."

—JUDY MAZEL, author of *The Beverly Hills Diet*

"Fat chance."

—GABE MIRKIN, skeptic

HISTORY won't know what to make of it.

In rich, enlightened twentieth-century America, why were people eating sowbelly scrapings, slaughterhouse waste, and seaweed? Why were they taking hormone shots made from the urine of pregnant women? Why were they starving themselves like Oriental mystics? Why were they stuffing themselves with grapes? Why were they offending one another with bad breath and gas?

The answer, future historians, is that it was all part of their compulsion to lose weight. Fat was their problem, and it made them desperate. If the "solution" meant throwing out common sense, they often seemed all too willing to do it.

These people were not dummies. Basically, they knew that the only real way to lose weight is to burn off more calories than one takes in. But that was the hard way. It took patience and self-denial, and sometimes even a drastic change in lifestyle.

So, people swarmed in droves to each new diet prophet who promised to make weight loss quick and painless. Their minds became garbage dumps for every fad diet on the market. So did their stomachs.

Some got thin.

Most got fat again.

Many hurt their health.

THE WORST OF THE FADS

For those of you who want a good diet, there are some excellent ones available. The good ones all have one thing in common: they're nutritionally balanced. They contain all forty-six nutrients. They also allow at least 1,300 calories a day, so you'll have enough energy to exercise.

There are some balanced diets that restrict you to 1,000 calories daily, but I don't recommend them. A thousand calories is sufficient only if you don't exercise. And as you already know, dieting without exercising drastically minimizes the odds that you'll maintain weight loss.

On the other hand, if you combine any good diet with a sound exercise program and some changes in bad habits, your chances of taking off weight and keeping it off are good.

Why, then, do so many people bypass the good diets in favor of useless or dangerous fad diets? Perhaps it's because there's nothing especially exotic or glamorous about the good ones. You don't see them in the tabloids or hear about them at the office. They can't compete with the fad diets for novel gimmicks, bloated promises, conversational value, or snob appeal. Moreover, the good diets seldom claim to be "miraculous" or "revolutionary" or based on some medical "breakthrough."

Often the fad diets are notable for their quasi-scientific approach. Many imply some new and special knowledge about the nature of food or the way your body uses it. Physicians and nutritionists can usually spot these claims for the claptrap they are. But an unwary public is often misled.

It's noteworthy that fad diets follow each other in such rapid succession. This may be explained by the fact that none of them works in the long run. A fad may catch on by producing quick, if brief, results. In the first flush of weight loss, dieters spread the word, and the diet's popularity grows. It fades as the dieters regain their weight and as bad side effects come to light. This readies the market for yet another fad, another phase in the disillusionment cycle.

The Beverly Hills Diet

This is one of the more recent big entries in the fad annals. Its author is Judy Mazel, an attractive and persuasive spokesperson with a boundless appetite for television talk shows. "I'm a born actress," she says. And indeed, her college training was in acting — not in medicine or nutrition.

It stands her in good stead as a book promoter, if not as a scientific specialist on obesity.

For the first ten days of the Mazel diet, you eat nothing but fruit — an exotic assortment that's easy to come by if you live in the tropics, California, or Florida. Of course, you get to eat quite a lot of fruit. Ms. Mazel says that five pounds of grapes a day are "not excessive."

On day eleven, you switch from fruits to starches. You get half a pound of bread for breakfast, with butter and three ears of corn to round out the day's menu. The diet goes on with an assortment of fruits, salads, and starches until day nineteen. Then, finally, you get some food that's a decent source of complete protein (steak or lobster).

FAT AS A "DIGESTIVE PROBLEM"

Ms. Mazel says that obesity is merely a digestive problem. "When your body doesn't process food, doesn't digest it, that food turns to fat," she states, adding that even noncaloric sweeteners and diet sodas turn to fat because they're "indigestible."

Having read the previous chapter of this book, you know that her assertions are completely contrary to the most basic scientific fact. Food you can't digest passes through your intestines without releasing calories. Therefore, it can't possibly be fattening. It's the food you *do* digest that can be stored as fat. As for artificial sweeteners and noncaloric drinks, they can't possibly turn to fat. They have few if any calories, and only calories create fat.

WEIGHT LOSS THROUGH DIARRHEA

There's a further irony in the Mazel diet. While proclaiming the virtues of "digestion," she puts you on a highly indigestible food.

The glut of fiber-rich fruits promotes diarrhea. Dr. Myron Winnick, director of the Institute of Human Nutrition at Columbia University, credits diarrhea with causing much of the weight loss the diet provides. He and other nutritionists have expressed alarm over this aspect of the diet. Ms. Mazel does not share their concern.

"If you have loose bowel movements, Hooray!" she says in her book. "Keep in mind that pounds leave you two main ways — bowel movements and urination. The more time you spend on the toilet, the better."

In fact, putting in time on the toilet with diarrhea and excessive urination is a very unhealthy and unsound approach to losing weight.

In the first place, most of the weight lost thereby is water, not fat.

Lost water may indeed equal lost pounds and even lost inches — but only for a very short time. Unless you want to court the dangers of dehydration, you'll quickly drink enough fluids to replace what you've lost. And when this happens, the pounds and inches return immediately. To lose weight in any meaningful sense, you have to lose fat, not water.

In the second place, excessive water loss can be dangerous. You already know how important a nutrient water is. You need it to maintain the integrity of every living cell in your body. You need it to maintain your blood volume and to help regulate your body temperature. You need a good supply of it to keep body minerals from becoming too concentrated. Mineral imbalances can disrupt your entire electrical system, including your heartbeat. In short, you need water to stay healthy and alive. Severe dehydration can kill you.

Even if you're only mildly dehydrated, you'll feel weak and tired. You'll have difficulty exercising. And if you try to exercise despite the weakness, you may develop a sudden rise in body temperature that will cause you to faint. Even if you don't try to exercise, the severe dehydration can eventually cause the extreme drop in blood pressure that constitutes shock.

A final point on Ms. Mazel's toilet touting: you don't lose body fat by excreting it. You lose it by expending it as energy.

Along with diarrhea, the bulky food on the Mazel diet tends to produce flatulence. Gas buildup can be uncomfortable, embarrassing, and terribly unchic, in Beverly Hills or anywhere else.

LOSING WEIGHT WITH ENZYMES?

Ms. Mazel reveals that the secret of her diet is understanding enzymes. She says that enzymes must work one at a time, never together, to break down food and thereby — according to her logic — keep the food from being fattening.

From what you learned about food and enzymes in the last chapter, you'll easily recognize this as another absurdity. Hardly any foods are nutritionally "pure." Almost all contain some carbohydrates, protein, and fat, regardless of which constituent predominates. Even Ms. Mazel's beloved grapes contain some fat and protein along with their carbohydrates.

Obviously, then, your enzymes have to work in concert. They're well accustomed to breaking down food by acting together, and they're perfectly able to do just that. If it were otherwise, nature would have chalked off mammals as a failed experiment long before man ever appeared on the scene. All the little critters would have starved to death through failure to absorb the food they ate.

HEALTH PROBLEMS WITH THE BEVERLY HILLS DIET

This diet can set you up for a host of difficulties. I've already enumerated the dangers of dehydration, which the diet promotes. It is also far too low in protein, so it can lead to lean-tissue breakdown. In addition, it encourages gorging by people who may already be compulsive in their eating habits.

But you have to hand it to Ms. Mazel. She thinks big. "I want to change the consciousness of the planet," she states. And to her many medical critics, she once replied in a magazine interview, "Sour grapes."

The Atkins Diet Revolution

One of the most controversial diet gurus of all is Dr. Robert Atkins, a New York physician. Dr. Atkins has been at war with much of the medical profession for years over whether his diet does or does not work, and whether it is or is not safe. He's been sued four times by patients who alleged that he damaged their health. He settled three cases out of court and successfully defended himself in the fourth.

If the Atkins diet were nutritionally sound, it would be a dieter's dream. As presented in his first book, *Dr. Atkins' Diet Revolution*, it allowed you to eat all the protein and fat you wanted. The trick was to eliminate or stringently limit carbohydrates.

Calories were no object. Dr. Atkins said you could eat 3,000, 4,000, 5,000 calories a day — whipped cream, steak, butter, mayonnaise, and many other rich goodies — and still lose weight.

Actually, the concept of the low-carbohydrate diet is far from revolutionary. It was first proposed about a century ago by a layman named William Banting. And Dr. Atkins is not its first prophet. One former one was Dr. Herman Taller with his much-criticized "Calories Don't Count" diet. Another was Dr. Irwin M. Stillman with his popular "Quick Weight Loss Diet."

Taller, Stillman, and Atkins contend that the way to lose weight is to deprive your body of carbohydrates so it will have to burn stored fat for energy. If you do this, they say, you'll mobilize your stored fat and burn it off.

Again, we have a theory based on the fallacy that the *source* of calories — not the calories themselves — is important. There is no scientific evidence to support this notion. If you take in fewer calories than you need, your body will indeed draw on its stored fat reserves for energy. But restricting carbohydrates will not make you burn the stored fat faster or more efficiently than restricting any other kind of food.

It is true that your body prefers to burn carbohydrates for energy during exercise. But eliminating the carbohydrates does not mean that you'll burn more stored fat during exercise. It simply means that you may not have the energy to exercise at all. And you could deprive your brain of its primary source of fuel, contributing to a feeling of fatigue and depletion.

In essence, then, the Atkins theory makes about as much sense as the idea that you should lie in bed all day to lose weight because the body burns fat rather than carbohydrates while at rest. Both notions violate the one and only equation governing weight: your weight rises or falls based on the *calorie* surplus or the *calorie* deficit you create.

Calories do indeed count. Calories are *all* that count. Gorging yourself on fat and protein will cause you only to accumulate more stored fat. It will do nothing to make you burn that fat at an accelerated rate.

WEIGHT LOSS THROUGH KETOSIS

The aim of the Atkins diet is to induce a state of *ketosis*, or high blood levels of ketones, in your body. You'll remember from Chapter 3 that ketones are chemical residues left behind when fat is burned for energy. They can be broken down to serve as a last-ditch fuel source, especially for your brain, if you're very low on carbohydrates or if you're starving. Dr. Atkins contends that ketones also help you lose weight by killing your appetite.

There's no hard scientific evidence that ketones suppress hunger directly, although they may curb your appetite by making you feel sick. Up to a point, ketones can be recycled for energy. But beyond that, they can build up in your bloodstream to make you feel weak and nauseated and give you a headache. The reason for this is that ketones are acids, and they make your blood more acid. Your body does not function well if blood-acid levels are abnormally high.

A far more pleasant way to suppress hunger is to exercise. Exercise will make you feel energetic instead of weak, and fit instead of sick. It will also help you burn more calories as an added bonus to inhibiting your hunger.

For most people, high ketone levels are more of a social handicap than a real health hazard. They cause bad breath. But if you're pregnant, or if you have any kidney ailment, they can pose a threat.

If you're pregnant, high blood acidity caused by ketones can damage the brain of your unborn child. As for your kidneys, they play a big role in getting rid of excess ketones. They break down some of them, and they eliminate others by allowing them to leave your body via your urine. If your kidneys aren't functioning properly, the acidic ketones can build up to dangerous, even toxic, levels in your blood. The high acidity can cause your brain to malfunction so that you become unconscious, or even die.

THE ATKINS DIET AND WATER LOSS

You have to urinate often to get rid of ketones. The Atkins diet promotes further water weight loss by restricting needed carbohydrates. The diet quickly depletes the sugar stored in your muscles and liver. Every gram of sugar they give up carries with it three grams of water.

This is why the Atkins diet can produce a dramatic weight loss in the first few days you're on it. Unfortunately, most of the loss is water. Unless you're careful to replace it, you risk getting dehydrated. And if water is all you've lost, replacing the water means replacing the weight.

If you escape feeling ill from ketosis and manage to follow the Atkins diet with gusto, water is all you're likely to lose. The diet's allowance of calories is theoretically unlimited, and an overabundance of calories from any kind of food ends up as body fat. I can't repeat it too often: losing weight means expending more calories than you take in. Once food is absorbed and the calorie costs of processing are paid, your body will store any surplus calories as body fat. It couldn't care less what kind of food you eat to create the surplus.

Dr. Atkins assumes that man is a carnivore. He is not. He's an omnivore. He was not meant to live by meat alone. If he tries to, he becomes subject to all the low-carbohydrate problems you have read about in Chapter 11.

The Lecithin, Kelp, B₆, and Vinegar Diet

A great fan of Dr. Atkins is Mary Ann Crenshaw, another best-selling author in the fad diet derby.

Ms. Crenshaw approves of inducing ketosis to lose weight. But to this method she adds a twist all her own in the form of her "Four Friends" — lecithin, kelp, vitamin B_6, and vinegar.

LECITHIN

"Pronounce it 'less-i-thin' and call it a miracle," Ms. Crenshaw exults over lecithin, an emulsifier found in mayonnaise and many salad dressings. This "miracle" is made from slaughterhouse waste and soybean extract. It's added to certain foods to keep their oil from settling out of suspension.

Lecithin enthusiasts contend that the substance behaves in your bloodstream much the same way it does in mayonnaise. It's supposed to keep your blood fat from settling out and plaquing up your artery walls. There's no evidence to support this notion, perhaps because blood is not, in fact, mayonnaise. Lecithin has no known special effect either on blood fat or any other kind of fat in your body.

Ms. Crenshaw also contends that lecithin is "full of vitamin E, the sexy shaper-upper." Another quaint notion. You need a certain small amount of vitamin E to help keep your cell membranes intact. This is what it does, and all it does, according to the best current medical research. A "sexy shaper-upper" it is not. And even if it were, eating lecithin wouldn't help. Lecithin is made up of several substances. But regardless of Ms. Crenshaw's enthusiasm, none of them is vitamin E.

KELP

Ms. Crenshaw's second "friend" is kelp, a kind of seaweed. She reasons that since kelp is rich in iodine, it might pep up your thyroid gland.

You'll remember from our discussion of hormones in Chapter 6 that the hormones that the thyroid gland secretes do help mobilize and burn stored fat. And the mineral iodine is, in fact, a constituent of them.

But it does not follow that overloading on iodine speeds up your thyroid gland in any way, shape, or form. It doesn't. Glands and hormones just aren't all that simple, and trying to manipulate them with special foods or additives is downright foolish. For a number of complicated medical reasons, overloading your system with iodine can even depress the production of thyroid hormones, giving you less instead of more.

Ms. Crenshaw says she takes six kelp tablets after every meal. She'd be better off eating seafood and using iodized salt, which give you all the iodine you need.

VITAMIN B₆ AND VINEGAR

As for vitamin B_6, Ms. Crenshaw says that 50 milligrams after every meal gave her quick and miraculous benefits in weight loss. Lord knows why. Vitamin B_6 figures in the metabolization of amino acids, not fat. It has nothing to do with getting rid of fat.

Ms. Crenshaw rounds out her medically nonsensical diet plan with this piquant piece of logic: "After all, oil and vinegar don't really mix. Maybe vinegar and my fat wouldn't either, and vinegar might just win out."

Vinegar wins out only in salad dressing. It's a kind of acetic acid that gets broken down into its basic components before it ever reaches your bloodstream — and certainly before it ever gets a chance to war with your stored fat. And the components of acetic acid have no fat-fighting properties whatever.

If Ms. Crenshaw stays thin on her diet, it's not because of help from her "friends." It's because she limits herself to 1,000 calories a day. This is the intake she reports, and it's certainly small enough to keep almost anyone sylphlike.

The Cellulite Diets

A number of these are in vogue. The most popular comes from Nicole Ronsard, who operates a beauty salon in New York City.

Cellulite is supposed to be made up of toxic body wastes that get trapped in pockets just under your skin, eluding your bloodstream's efforts to flush them out. Supposedly, these nasty little deposits fill up with water and pooch out, creating the dimpling you may see on fat parts of your body — your hips, thighs, and upper arms, for instance.

But cellulite is not ordinary fat, say Ms. Ronsard and the others, and ordinary diets won't cure it. You need special diets, along with special exercises. In addition, you must poke, prod, pinch, rub, and otherwise discourage cellulite by attacking it from the outside.

The Ronsard diet relies heavily on fruits and vegetables, with meat, fish, and poultry in sparing amounts. This is acceptable enough. The problem with the diet is its object. It does battle with an imaginary enemy.

It's true that cellulite is no ordinary fat problem, nor any other kind of problem, since it doesn't exist. There is no such thing as "cellulite." Dimpling in the skin is caused by excess fat — no more, no less. Tiny ligaments run from your skin through the fat underneath to the underlying layer of muscle. If you have too much fat, it pokes up between the ligaments, causing tiny bulges. You can rub and pummel all you want, but they won't go away. If you lose enough fat, they will.

Depending on how your fat is distributed, the dimpling may persist in some areas longer than in others as you lose weight. But fat can be lost only from areas where it is stored. So eventually, the excess fat that causes the dimpling should diminish enough to eliminate the dimples.

Exercise can help. Along with being essential to healthy and lasting weight loss, exercise helps firm your muscles. As weight loss shrinks the fat layer and brings the muscles closer to the skin surface, the firmer muscles will help give you a smooth and attractive look.

CELLULITE AND NIACIN

Some cellulite gurus recommend taking massive doses of niacin, one of the B vitamins. Since niacin helps dilate your blood vessels, they reason, it helps your bloodstream reach the cellulite and wash it away.

Aside from being useless, massive doses of niacin can be dangerous. Potential side effects include flushing and itching of the skin, blood-sugar problems, gout, ulcers, and liver damage.

The Fructose Diets

There are several of these, among them *Dr. Cooper's Fabulous Fructose Diet*, by physician J.T. Cooper. (Dr. Atkins is also a fructose fan.)

These diets propose that the basic sweetener in your diet should be fructose, not sucrose. Sucrose is ordinary granulated table sugar, made up of glucose and fructose. Fructose is also a component of honey. Since fructose diets have created a demand for it, it's also available commercially now in a pure form.

Fructose advocates contend that their sugar helps keep your blood-sugar levels steady, while glucose makes them bounce up and down. They maintain that by keeping blood-sugar levels steady, fructose also helps keep insulin levels steady. As you know, a low and even flow of insulin discourages fat deposition.

To understand this misleading theory, you must first recall how your body processes carbohydrates. You learned in Chapter 11 that glucose and fructose are both single sugars. But while glucose can pass through your liver unchanged, fructose must be intercepted and converted to glucose before the liver releases it for general circulation in your blood.

Since it requires an extra step in processing, fructose does enter your bloodstream more gradually than glucose. If you measure the difference in a laboratory, you'll find that, indeed, blood-sugar and insulin levels are slightly higher in response to glucose than they are to fructose.

But unless you're a laboratory rat, the difference is so small that it has no meaning whatever. Healthy people who eat normally do not have steep peaks and valleys in blood-sugar levels, or in insulin responses, no matter what kind of sugar they eat — glucose and fructose together (table sugar) or pure fructose.

HYPOGLYCEMIA

And now a word about what must be the most overdiscussed, overdramatized, and overdiagnosed disease in America. *Hypoglycemia* is an ailment in which blood-sugar levels are abnormally and dangerously low. Its symptoms include a rapid pulse, shakiness, an empty feeling in the stomach, cold sweats, and a feeling of impending doom. Extreme anxiety or fear can produce the same symptoms.

There is also something called *rebound hypoglycemia*. This involves an abnormal response to eating sugar in which the victim's blood-sugar levels rise precipitously and then drop to hypoglycemic levels.

If you suffer from either kind of hypoglycemia, the choice between eating table sugar or eating fructose should be the last thing on your mind. Hypoglycemia can be a symptom of something much worse. If you suffer from it, you should get checked for a possible brain tumor, liver disease, or hormonal abnormality.

In fact, however, hypoglycemia is a very rare disease, affecting perhaps one person in 10,000. It seems common because it has somehow become a catchall explanation for symptoms that usually are more properly ascribed to psychological problems, such as severe anxiety.

Fructose mavens contend that fructose helps protect you from hypoglycemia — a dubious contention in itself. But since the disease is so rare, protection from it is about as valuable as protection against getting hit by a meteor. Damage from either one is highly unlikely.

FRUCTOSE AND MUSCLE ENERGY

The backup argument for fructose fans is that your muscles can use it directly for quick energy. Glucose can enter the muscles only with a push from insulin, while fructose can get in on its own.

The problem here is that fructose never circulates to the muscles as fructose. The liver converts it to glucose before it goes into your general blood circulation. So if you want to get fructose directly into your muscles, you have to inject it. Since most of you aren't sitting around with a hypodermic needle to go with your morning coffee, this won't do you much good.

Glucose and fructose are both sugars. They are both dense sources of calories. They both cause an insulin response — a response that for all practical purposes is about the same.

My advice is to forget the whole controversy and consider the advantages of a noncaloric sugar substitute. It can't make you fat, and it will affect your blood-sugar and insulin levels insignificantly (more about the noncaloric sugar substitute saccharin in the next chapter).

The Last Chance Diet

This liquid protein regimen holds the record as the most destructive fad of all. For some people, it was indeed the "last chance." While on the diet, they died.

The Last Chance Diet was the title of a book by Dr. Robert Linn, an osteopath from Broomall, Pennsylvania. The diet was based on a concoction invented by Dr. Linn and called "Prolinn." He described it as "a formula composed of all the amino acids needed to form a protein molecule." In the late 1970s, Prolinn was all the rage.

Prolinn is derived from beef hides and the underbellies of sows. At first it was available only from doctors. Later it became a hot over-the-counter item, selling for about $14 a quart. Most druggists loved it. A sellout item itself, it also promoted sales of vitamin and mineral supplements recommended by Dr. Linn to go with it. The supplements were potassium, folic acid, vitamin C, and a vitamin and mineral multiple.

"Protein-Sparing Fasting"

Dr. Linn called his diet a "protein-sparing fast." For most people, the fast meant taking two tablespoons of Prolinn several times a day, totaling a near-starvation intake of about 420 calories. Along with the liquid and the pills, you were supposed to drink two and a half quarts a day of water and other noncaloric fluids.

By "protein-sparing," Dr. Linn meant that his diet could put you on a bare minimum of calories without causing you to lose lean-muscle tissue. It was supposed to give you the quick weight loss of a total fast, but without the risks.

In fact, this claim was not true.

In the first place, Prolinn was not a "complete" protein supplement. It had only seven of the nine essential amino acids. Your lean tissue is constantly breaking down and releasing its amino acids, as you learned in the last chapter, and it needs all nine essential amino acids to renew itself properly.

Even if it had been complete, Prolinn could not have prevented lean-tissue breakdown entirely. Study after study shows that diets consisting only of massive doses of protein can't do that. If you aren't getting complete, balanced, and adequate nutrition, the tissue that makes up your muscles and your vital organs—including your heart—begins to deteriorate. A prolonged stint on a protein-only diet at near-starvation levels can kill you.

Prolinn Consumers—and Victims

Despite the dangers, thousands of people were lured by the hope of the quick and massive weight loss the Linn plan offered. Business boomed. The doctor opened a number of branch offices. At their height, these branch offices were treating more than 1,500 patients a day. The patients paid $100 for their first visit and $60 for each weekly visit thereafter. This entitled them to weekly checkups and weekly doles of Prolinn and supplements.

Dr. Linn advised that his diet should only be followed under a doctor's supervision, a common caveat for diets. Few people heeded the warning. The diet plan and its raw materials were easy to get and simple to use.

The Prolinn program did produce staggering weight losses for some people. Most regained the weight after abandoning the fast. In any case, the price tag on some of those lost pounds was horrendous.

The U.S. Food and Drug Administration has documented at least fifty-eight cases of people dying while on the Prolinn diet. In addition, the U.S. Center for Disease Control did a sobering study on women who relied on liquid protein as their main source of calories for more than two months. The government scientists found a health-risk pattern they described as follows:

"This pattern is characterized by either sudden death or death due to intractable cardiac arrhythmias in individuals with no previous history of heart disease."

Fortunately, liquid protein diets like the Prolinn diet are waning in popularity. Nevertheless, some desperate souls still try them. They shouldn't, and neither should you.

DEFICIENCY DIETS

The preceding diets may be remarkable for their dangers and/or absurdities. But they're by no means the only bad diets around. I can't overstress that any diet that's deficient in any nutrient poses a potential health hazard.

Note that I said a "potential" hazard. Being deficient in even a single nutrient can eventually cause problems ranging from chipped fingernails to cancer. But most reducing diets aren't going to make you seriously deficient in anything unless you stay on them too long.

This is partly because your body is a remarkably durable and flexible mechanism. It's also partly because so few foods are nutritionally pure, as you've already seen. For instance, you may go on a high-fiber diet that allows you no visible fat at all. But you'll get most, if not all, the fat you need from the small amounts found in whole grains.

Still, you're going to get sick on a deficiency diet if you stay on it too long, especially if that diet is a fast or is very low in calories. Remember: to get adequate amounts of all the nutrients you need, you must have at least 1,300 calories a day if you exercise, and 1,000, calories a day if you don't. Diets allowing fewer calories are depriving you of one or more nutrients. Avoid them.

In the last chapter, you learned why a balanced diet is essential to your health. Let's briefly review and expand a bit on the dangers each kind of lopsided diet may present:

Low-Carbohydrate Diets

The Atkins and the Prolinn diets are extreme examples of this kind. Other popular entries, though less extreme, include the Complete Scarsdale Medical Diet, by Dr. Herman Tarnower; the Doctor's Quick Weight Loss Diet, by Dr. Stillman; the Woman Doctor's Diet for Women, by Dr. Barbara Edelstein, and the "Drinking Man's Diet" of the mid 1960s.

Diets too low in carbohydrates can make you dehydrated, dangerously ketotic, and too tired to exercise. They can cause damage to fetuses, since unborn babies cannot use ketones and depend entirely on glucose to nourish their brains. They can pose a hazard to people with diseased or malfunctioning kidneys. You're already acquainted with all these dangers.

In addition, a diet very low in carbohydrates can make you subject to gout. When you're ketotic, the uric acid normally eliminated by your kidneys has to compete with ketones. As the ketones are eliminated instead of the uric acid, the uric acid builds up in your bloodstream. If its levels get too high, it can precipitate out of your bloodstream and crystallize in your joints, causing severe pain. This is gout.

Finally, this kind of diet may make you yo-yo. A low-carbohydrate regimen is hard to stay on. The weakness and the sick feeling ketosis can cause are very unpleasant. As a result, the temptation to abandon the diet is very great. As you return to your old eating patterns, you regain weight.

Water loss and an appetite dampened by ketosis may produce dramatic short-term results on a low-carbohydrate diet. But usually these are only precursors of rapid and dangerous regain. There is no medical evidence that low-carbohydrate diets produce permanent weight loss for most people.

Low-Carbohydrate and High-Protein Diets

Low-carbohydrate diets and high-protein diets are usually one and the same. Obviously, if you're eating less of one thing, you're probably eating more of something else. Since fat is the most fattening of the three calorie-bearing nutrient groups, almost all reducing diets juggle the proportions of the remaining two, carbohydrates and protein.

However, high protein brings its own set of problems to a low-carbohydrate diet:

- Monotony. Such a diet centers either on protein supplements or on a tedious round of poultry, meat, and fish.
- Potential kidney damage. Remember, your body can't store protein. It converts the excess into ammonia and organic acids and eliminates them through your urine. On a diet very low in carbohydrates and very high in protein, your kidneys must work overtime to process ketones and cope with water loss from sugar depletion. Protein-breakdown products overtax them still further. Ailing kidneys can suffer or even fail under the strain.
- Aggravated dehydration. The same principle involved in the point I just made applies here. On a very low-carbohydrate diet, you're losing water two ways: from ketosis and from sugar depletion. A diet that's also very high in protein adds a third factor to the dehydration problem. Ammonia and organic acids from protein breakdown must be eliminated in your urine. So urination becomes even more frequent. The ammonia and organic acids also add to the competition your uric acid is already getting from ketones, so the threat of gout increases.
- Calcium loss. Protein tends to draw the mineral calcium out of your system. In great excess, protein can eventually cause your bones to soften.

High-protein, low-carbohydrate diets are going out of style, although they enjoyed a long reign of great popularity.

Low-Carbohydrate and High-Fat Diets

This kind of diet is very rare, since it is necessarily high in calories. The only example of note was the original version of the Atkins diet, which allowed unlimited fat.

It's fortunate that this sort of diet is a rarity. It has the potential to elevate low-density cholesterol levels in the blood. This increases the risk of cardiovascular disease such as hardening of the arteries, strokes, and heart attacks.

Low Protein

In swinging away from the high-protein diet concept, the diet fad pendulum may have gone too far in the other direction. The Beverly Hills Diet is the most popular example of one that is far too low in protein.

A diet too low in protein can cause the breakdown of your lean tissue, beginning with your skin, hair, and nails. If you persist long enough in a diet very low in both calories and protein, you can kill yourself. Your heart and other vital organs eventually grow too weak to function.

Aside from water loss, more than 50 percent of the weight you lose on a low-protein diet will be from muscle tissue. If you then regain the weight through overeating, all of it will be in the form of fat. With this scenario, you end up worse than you started. Even at the same net weight, you'll have less muscle and more fat.

Still, a diet that's low in protein and high in carbohydrates is usually safer than one with the combination in reverse. The carbohydrates satisfy your energy requirements, so your body doesn't have to call on its own lean tissue for fuel. Besides, you need comparatively little protein, as long as you're getting the right kind — protein with all nine essential amino acids.

Low Fat

Most low-calorie diets bill themselves as low fat, but this is seldom truly the case. If the diet allows you animal protein, you're getting plenty of fat. Even the leanest meats contain some fat, as do eggs and all dairy products. Similarly, high-carbohydrate diets provide fat from whole grains.

Only fasts — true fasts and the protein-supplement variations — are low fat in the sense of being fat-deficient, and these are dangerous.

A truly fat-free diet can make you deficient in fat-soluble vitamins. If it prevents your getting enough vitamin A, it can interfere with your immune system. If this happens, you're at greater risk for various infections and a variety of cancers.

A fat-deficient diet can also deprive you of the linoleic acid you need to help you build cell membranes and sex hormones. Since fat helps you absorb certain minerals, a very low-fat diet that's also low in minerals can cause problems.

LOW FAT AND THE PRITIKIN DIET

The Pritikin Diet, which gained many converts in the 1970s, is very high in complex carbohydrates and very low in fat. It has merit as a high-energy, high-fiber program, and certainly it is head and shoulders above the fad diets I've been discussing. However, some critics contend the diet is dangerously low in fat.

Nathan Pritikin is an inventor who got interested in nutrition some years ago while fighting his own problems with high cholesterol. He devised a diet that has since been refined and tested at his Longevity Institute in California. He contends the diet cured his own health problems and that it can contribute to health and long life for most people.

Sincere, well-meaning, and knowledgeable, Mr. Pritikin has attracted a great many followers — and some critics. He replies to criticism of his diet by pointing to the fact that the whole grains, fruits, vegetables, and vitamin D–enriched skim milk in his diet provide and help process all the essential vitamins you need for health.

Mr. Pritikin's defense of his theory is fairly persuasive. However, there is one potentially serious problem with the Pritikin Diet — the possibility of mineral deficiency.

As you know, fat helps you absorb minerals. Fiber decreases absorption. Theoretically, then, the Pritikin Diet could cause you to run low on certain minerals, particularly calcium. Over the years, this could lead to bone softening. Since this problem can take as long as twenty years to appear, there are no studies yet to show that the Pritikin plan is absolutely safe in regard to minerals.

In any case, the Pritikin Diet can be tough to follow in the real world. It calls for you to eat four pounds of food a day in eight meals. This means you have to go around with a bag of vegetables in tow.

Fasting and Mini-Calorie Diets

Fasting can be fatal.

There's the perfectly obvious danger that if you fast long enough, you'll starve to death. Hardly anyone, no matter how fat when the fast begins, can survive more than seventy days without food.

However, you can die much sooner than that from mineral imbalances. While fasting, you lose minerals rapidly through urination, and you don't replace them. A mineral imbalance can lead to irregular heartbeats that can be lethal.

Since fasting is the total deficiency diet, it can cause every deficiency problem I've mentioned thus far. It's unquestionably dangerous. *Don't do it.*

Some adherents advocate occasional limited fasts, such as one or two foodless days each week or each month. The theory goes that aside from helping you control your weight, this kind of fasting rests your system and "cleans you out." There's no scientific basis for such claims. In fact, there's no known medical benefit whatever that derives from fasting.

THE SCARSDALE DIET
Very low-calorie diets are less dangerous than fasting, but still dangerous enough. "Very low" means fewer than 1,000 calories per day. Liquid protein diets and several other crash programs fall into this category. So do some diets regarded by many people as more sensible, such as the Scarsdale Medical Diet. Scarsdale gives you between 750 and 1,000 calories a day. Its author, the late Dr. Herman Tarnower, was not a quack but a respected cardiologist who understood nutrition. No doubt this is why he recommended that dieters follow his regimen for only two weeks at a time, alternating it with a plan that allowed more calories, mostly in the form of carbohydrates. Like other very low-calorie diets, however, the Scarsdale Diet is, at best, a temporary measure against overweight — it is not a diet that can be followed permanently, over a long period, and it will not change the eating habits that result in the dieter's yo-yo syndrome of rapid loss, rapid regaining.

THE I LOVE NEW YORK DIET
Another, more recent, representative of the "alternating plan" school of dieting is the I Love New York Diet, by consumer advocate Bess Myerson and Bill Adler, a literary agent. The I Love New York Diet — so called because it is based on a weight-loss program that was originally developed for the New York City Health Department — has a gimmick: for one week you go on a very low-calorie crash diet (600 to 800 calories a day), after which you are rewarded by a week in which you are allowed to consume 1,800 calories a day. The idea is that dieting will be pleasanter if the dieter is allowed to relieve the agony of a semistarvation diet with a binge every other week.

The problem, of course, is that this system can't work in the long run — alternating very low-calorie weeks with more permissive ones simply sets you up for the yo-yo pattern again. People who have more than just a few pounds to shed are as unlikely to keep them off successfully on this diet as they were on the Scarsdale Diet.

THE ZEN MACROBIOTIC DIET
One of the most notorious mini-calorie diets of recent years was the Zen Macrobiotic Diet. This quasi-mystical regimen was an insult to true

Buddhists, who frown on food fads. It required the dieter to reduce food intake in six drastic stages, ending up with nothing but tea and brown rice. Several people died on this diet.

You can lose lean tissue rapidly on a mini-calorie diet, and you can suffer mineral imbalances and vitamin deficiencies that may prove harmful or even fatal. Such diets often provide very rapid weight loss — followed by equally rapid gain.

In addition, many studies show a high incidence of depression, irritability, and even suicide associated with mini-calorie diets. Coordination and concentration are impaired. Students eating too little may do badly in school, and workers show diminished job performance.

THE CAMBRIDGE DIET

The Cambridge Diet is a gift to us from England, which nevertheless remains an ally. This diet poses the same danger as any mini-calorie crash diet. It can cause you to lose lean tissue, including heart tissue, and it has doubtful value for lasting weight loss.

With this diet plan, you get all your calories for the first four weeks from a beverage. The exact recipe for this drink has not been made public. But its manufacturers say it contains the recommended daily allowances for all essential vitamins and some minerals, as well as carbohydrates and protein, for a total of 330 calories per drink.

Staying on the Cambridge Diet for one month probably won't hurt the normal dieter. But anyone with a weak heart could lose a dangerous amount of heart-muscle tissue in this time. In fact, doctors have reported cases of patients on the Cambridge Diet who suffered irregular heartbeats.

Prompted by the FDA, sellers of the diet recommend that you not stay on the beverage alone for more than four consecutive weeks. After that, you continue drinking the beverage — at a cost of about $17.50 a week — but you supplement it with food. This regimen is intended to be lifelong.

With an intake of only 330 calories a day, almost anyone will lose weight fast in the early stages of the Cambridge Diet. But the dieter is not likely to learn good eating and exercise habits in one month, or to become so attached to the Cambridge elixir that it is an acceptable substitute for one's favorite food.

The diet is fairly new, but don't be surprised to hear that its adherents who enjoyed early success are yo-yoing upward again.

Skipping Meals

There are diets that recommend skipping lunch, diets that recommend skipping dinner, and diets that recommend eating nothing after a certain hour each day.

The problem with all these diets is that they encourage you to eat a few large meals instead of many small ones. As you learned in Chapter 6, frequent eating is much better for you than limiting your meals, as long as you're not taking in more calories. Small meals bring on only small insulin responses. They also encourage maximum calorie-burning activity by your brown fat.

One noteworthy meal-skipping diet was proposed by two physicians, Drs. William F. Kremer and Laura Kremer. They recommend skipping breakfast. They contend that a 400-calorie lunch and 500-calorie dinner are plenty to see the dieter through until lunch the next day.

I thoroughly disagree. Since your liver stores only a twelve-hour supply of sugar, there's a chance that your brain will run low on fuel if you skip breakfast. You need breakfast, or at least brunch, to ward off mid-morning fatigue and weakness.

There is No Such Thing as a Safe Reducing Diet that Contains Fewer than 400 Calories a Day

A study of seventeen people who died while dieting showed that their hearts degenerated in the same way as in starvation. Eating complete protein, taking potassium supplements and vitamins, and having medical supervision did not protect them (see H. E. Sours, et al., *American Journal of Clinical Nutrition* 34 [1981]: 453).

When you lose weight rapidly by any means, as much as 50 percent of your weight loss can come from loss of muscle. Since your heart is a muscle, it can become so small that it will be too weak to pump blood through your body. You can develop an irregular heartbeat and die.

The safest, most pleasant way to lose weight is to lose it slowly through adequate diet and exercise.

Additive Diets

Dieter beware. Additive diets are those that claim some special benefit from eating a particular food or taking some special supplement. You'll remember, for instance, Ms. Crenshaw's lecithin, vinegar, vitamin B_6, and kelp. Then there's Dr. Cooper's fructose, and the niacin of the anticellulite crusaders.

A hormone called *human chorionic gonadotropin*, or *HCG*, also deserves mention in this group.

HCG was introduced as a weight-loss medication by a British-born doctor named Albert T. Simeons, who first used it in India. HCG is a form of growth hormone produced by the human placenta and extracted from the urine of pregnant women.

Dr. Simeons contended that HCG mobilized stored fat for energy burnoff. With this fuel source available, he said, a dieter could subsist healthily and happily on only 500 calories a day. The HCG was supposed to suppress hunger while it was melting off fat.

At one time, HCG was the most widespread obesity medication administered in the United States. Some doctors liked it because it assured them of a steady clientele. Patients had to come in once a week for an injection of the hormone.

The patients lost weight, which is not surprising. Anyone will lose weight on a starvation-level diet of 500 calories a day. However, there was no evidence linking the weight loss directly to the HCG. After investigating Dr. Simeons's theory, the Food and Drug Administration said in 1975 that HCG was, in itself, ineffective as a weight-loss tool. The government scientists found no evidence that it quieted hunger or helped melt away or redistribute fat.

NO MAGIC ELIXIR

How did people endure the rigors of the HCG diet? Probably they managed because the gimmick gave them a focus for the hope, faith, and desperation that mark the chronic fad dieter.

There's hardly a fat person alive who doesn't wish for some magic pill, powder, or potion that will painlessly lift off the extra pounds. Unfortunately, there is no such thing. No hormone, no vitamin or mineral, no drug or special food has ever been proven uniquely potent for weight reduction.

Some eminent researchers, including Dr. Albert Stunkard of the University of Pennsylvania, believe that science will someday find a final biochemical cure for obesity. This may well be, and we all hope for it. But this doesn't mean we should look for it or wait for it. It hasn't happened yet, nor is it on the near horizon.

13.

THE GETTING THIN DIET

So now you're a walking encyclopedia of bad diets. Where does that leave you?

It leaves you in search of a *good* diet, of course. Take heart; I'm about to give you one.

I make no claim that the Getting Thin Diet is the *only* good diet in existence. But it does offer a pleasant, uncomplicated approach to good eating, based on sound medical facts about nutrition and physiology. And while I offer neither magic nor miracles, I can make you two promises:

- Those of you who follow the Getting Thin Diet will look, feel, and *be* healthy. The diet offers complete and well-balanced nutrition at a calorie cost geared to a tangible weight loss.
- Those of you who stay with the diet's principles, in combination with a good exercise program, will lose all the weight you want, and you will keep it off for life.

WHAT A GOOD DIET DOES

The Getting Thin Diet works because it does the things a good weight-loss diet must do:

- It protects your health by giving you all the nutrients you need.
- It gives you enough calories to allow you to exercise effectively — 1,300 calories a day.
- It is nevertheless low enough in calories to create the systematic calorie deficit you need for optimum weight loss. You will lose *fast* enough to maintain your determination and enthusiasm. But you will lose *gradually* enough to maximize your chances of staying thin permanently.
- It teaches you good eating habits. The Getting Thin Diet will enable you

not only to lose weight without suffering, but also to learn the principles of proper eating and incorporate them into your lifestyle while you lose weight. And you follow them for a lifetime to keep the weight off.

- It is flexible. You use the principles of the Getting Thin Diet to construct a personalized diet for yourself — one that is expressly tailored to your own tastes and needs. The foods can vary widely and still not violate the principles of effective, controlled weight loss.

How Much Will You Lose?

With the Getting Thin Diet, you will lose about 2 pounds a week. Some people may lose around 3 pounds a week.

Q. I can lose about $2^1/_2$ pounds a week on reducing diets, without exercise. But those diets only allowed me 1,000 calories a day. Why do I get more on this diet?

A. You need the additional 300 calories on the Getting Thin Diet in order to exercise. The additional 300 calories represent the minimum amount of energy needed to supply your muscles with sugar as fuel for exercise. The higher calorie level also ensures that you will be getting all the other nutrients you need for good health.

Q. But won't I lose less weight on a 1,300–calorie diet?

A. No — not if you exercise. The moderate exercise I recommend in Chapters 15 and 16 will burn off the additional 300 calories a day. The net result as far as weight loss goes will be about the same as if you were on a 1,000–calorie diet.

Q. Then why not just forget about exercise and stay on a 1,000–calorie diet?

A. Because, as you already know from previous chapters, exercise is vital to the dieter who wants to lose weight and not regain it. Exercise heightens the calorie-burning power of your metabolism and controls your appestat. It also makes you look and feel better — and that sense of physical well-being is a huge psychological plus when you're dieting. You will actually find dieting physically *easier* when you are on a moderate exercise program — not harder.

Q. Will I lose weight on the Getting Thin Diet if I *don't* exercise?

A. Yes — though more slowly. Thirteen hundred calories are about 500 calories a day fewer than most people need to maintain their bodies and fuel their muscle movement through an ordinary nonexercise day. Since a pound of fat represents 3,500 calories, you should lose about a pound a week even without exercise.

But although you can use the diet without exercise, I urge you not to. As I have stressed time and time again, *no* diet is likely to give you lasting results unless you exercise along with it, because exercise enhances body processes that help protect you against the yo-yo syndrome. And it is essential if you want to keep up a steady, easily measurable rate of weight loss that will help you feel you are getting closer to your goal.

Q. Well, in that case, wouldn't it be smart to go on a 1,000–calorie diet and exercise at the same time? I'd probably lose even faster than on 1,300 calories.

A. Sorry — the answer to that one is no. It is true that you would, in effect, be putting yourself on a 700–calorie a day diet, but, for reasons not fully understood, your average weekly weight loss would not be appreciably greater. All you would do would be to exhaust yourself and probably harm your health — that's assuming that you could stick with such a low-energy diet long enough to do so.

LOSING WEIGHT SLOWLY

What all this boils down to is that *to lose weight permanently, you must lose it slowly.* The 1,300 calories a day are what you need to be able to lose weight steadily, exercise, and have plenty of mental and physical energy from the nutrients your body requires.

Also, because you will lose weight slowly, you'll lose more fat and less muscle. People who lose more than 5 pounds of weight a week on semi-starvation crash diets often lose as much as 50 percent of their weight in muscle tissue. On the other hand, a slow-loss diet results in far more lost fat than muscle. If you exercise while you're losing weight, you may even gain muscle.

Finally, *you are more likely to keep the weight off.* Innumerable studies point up an inescapable flaw in crash dieting: the weight lost fastest is the weight regained fastest. Diets that cause rapid weight loss are extremely difficult to follow over a period of months, and virtually impossible over a period of years. Can you imagine taking in only 800 calories a day forever? Or spending the rest of your life fasting on a regular basis? Or eating only fruit as long as you live? Of course not.

Besides, if you lose weight very quickly, you don't give yourself time to develop new and lasting attitudes toward food and new patterns of eating and exercise.

You need a new lifestyle, not just a new diet, and new lifestyles take time to develop. Take that time, and your patience will be rewarded with lasting results.

THE GETTING THIN DIET
The Five Food Groups

The foods you are allowed on the Getting Thin Diet consist of five groups. The groups are based on an excellent program originally developed by the U.S. Department of Agriculture in the 1950s and improved since then, which organizes foods according to their predominant nutritional values. The five food groups are:

• Group 1: *Meats, Fish, Poultry, Eggs, Cheeses, Legumes*

   This group includes most foods very high in protein, the main source for amino acids. Meat, fish, poultry, eggs, and cheese supply all the nine essential amino acids. These foods (especially red meat) also are excellent sources of the B vitamins and iron. Eggs provide vitamins A and D; cheese offers vitamins B_2 and B_{12} and calcium.

   Legumes — beans, dry peas, nuts — supply many of the essential amino acids. In combination with grains and cereals or with animal proteins, they supply all nine.

   This group also supplies some fat, which you need to function properly.

• Group 2: *Grains, Cereals, Starchy Vegetables (Corn, Potatoes, etc.)*

   These foods are great sources of carbohydrates, which you need for muscle fuel and energy. Grains and cereals also supply almost all of the B vitamins, vitamin E, and some iron and protein.

• Group 3: *Vegetables and Fruits*

   Vegetables and fruits are the other great source of carbohydrates. Leafy vegetables, such as spinach, lettuce, cabbage, and celery, are rich in fiber to prevent constipation and to fill you up with a minimum of calories. Except for avocados, almost all fruits and vegetables have a low caloric density, because much of their bulk is made up of fiber and water. For this reason, they are on the whole the least fattening foods you can eat.

   Dark green vegetables, deep yellow vegetables, and a number of fruits are good sources of vitamin A. Dark green vegetables also give you high amounts of vitamin B_2, folic acid, iron, and magnesium. Certain vegetables, such as collard, kale, mustard, and turnips, contain calcium. Yellow vegetables offer thiamine, riboflavin, and niacin.

Vitamins B_1, B_6, and C, as well as iron, are abundant in certain fruits and their juices (oranges, grapefruits, lemons, strawberries, and pineapples are all high-vitamin fruits). These vitamins are also found in cantaloupes, tomatoes, broccoli, and brussels sprouts. Citrus fruits are a good source of folic acid, while bananas are rich in potassium. And sixteen or more trace minerals are found in most vegetables and in many fruits as well.

• Group 4: *Milk*

Milk — whole, skim, and yogurt — is a rich source of protein, calcium, vitamin A, and vitamins B_2 and B_{12}. Most milk is fortified with vitamin D.

Because milk is such an excellent source of essential nutrients, it is very important that you take the full amount allowed on the Getting Thin Diet: 2 servings each day. Bear in mind, however, that whole milk is heavy in fat, and ice cream, though allowed in small amounts on the Diet, is heavy in sugar as well. I therefore strongly recommend that you learn to substitute fat-free skim milk for whole or "low-fat" milk.

• Group 5: *Fats and Oils*

This group includes butter, margarine, oils, most nuts, mayonnaise, animal fats, salad dressings. It provides vitamins A and E (in oil), and vitamin B_1, pantothenic acid, and biotin (in nuts). Most important, fats provide linoleic acid, the only fatty acid your body can't manufacture.

As you know, it is recommended that you cut back on your intake of *all* fat, to less than 30 percent of the total. The Getting Thin Diet provides you with a fat intake closer to this ideal than what you've probably been getting. And, if you prefer to cut down on saturated fats, choose those on the list for Group 5 that are not asterisked (these are unsaturated). I have also suggested prudent limits for foods high in exogenous cholesterol, such as eggs, red meats, and organ meats. But *do not* omit the permitted quantities of fats from your diet. Remember, you need a certain level of fat in your intestines to absorb the fat-soluble vitamins and keep your immune system functioning well.

• *Minimal Calories*

This group, included in the Getting Thin Diet, consists of foods that are so low in calories that they do not need to be measured if taken in normal quantities.

Counting Calories

Organization of the Getting Thin Diet by the food groups means that following it is like ordering meals in a Chinese restaurant. In other words, you choose one item for one category of food, a second from the next category, and so on. You do not have to count calories unless you wish to, because they have already been counted for you in the serving portions I specify. To get about 1,300 calories daily, just select one food from each of the different groups. Such selecting ensures that you will have a diet close to the ideal proportions of about 15 percent protein, 60 percent carbohydrates, and 25 percent fat, containing all the vitamins and minerals you need.

"Aha," I hear you experienced calorie-counters out there muttering, "he says, 'about 1,300.'" That's right. Since some foods — red meats, hard cheeses, or legumes — are relatively more fattening than foods like fish or low-fat cheeses, your calorie intake will differ somewhat from day to day. On some days you may consume only 1,100 calories, while on others you might go higher than 1,300. As long as you get about 1,300 calories a day as a weekly average by choosing prudently from both ends of the calorie range, this variation will not affect your overall weight loss.

Of course, if you wish, you can plan you daily menus to work out to exactly 1,300 calories every time. Furthermore, if you are a first-time dieter or someone who is unfamiliar with the caloric vlues of common foods, count calories as long as you want to lose weight, in order to make yourself more conscious of how many calories you are consuming.

HOW THE GETTING THIN DIET WORKS

On the Getting Thin Diet, you eat a fixed number of premeasured servings from the major food groups every day. The key word for this diet is *serving*. The foods you may select from each group, along with their serving sizes, are listed on pages 167–176.

Here's how it works:

1. Look at the Plan, below. There you'll see how many servings from each group you can have for each main meal or snack.

2. Now, turn to the lists that begin on page 167. Here you will see what foods you can choose from each category. To the left of each food

The Diet Plan

• **BREAKFAST**

Group 1 (Meats): 1 serving
Group 2 (Grains and Cereals): 1 serving
Group 3 (Vegetables and Fruits): 1 fruit serving
Group 4 (Milk): $1/_2$ serving*
Group 5 (Fats and Oils): 1 serving
Group 6 (Minimal Calories): Beverage and seasonings

• **MIDMORNING SNACK**

Group 4 (Milk): $1/_2$ serving*
Group 6 (Minimal Calories): Fat-free broth with seasonings, or other beverages and
    seasonings from this list (optional)

• **LUNCH**

Group 1 (Meats): 2 servings
Group 2 (Grains and Cereals): 2 servings
Group 3 (Vegetables and Fruits): 1 vegetable serving from List A
Group 5 (Fats and Oils): 1 serving
Group 6 (Minimal Calories): Beverage and seasonings

• **AFTERNOON SNACK**

Group 3 (Vegetables and Fruits): 1 vegetable serving from List A (optional)
                                  1 fruit serving
Group 6 (Minimal Calories): Fat-free broth with seasonings or other beverages and
    seasonings from this list (optional)

• **DINNER**

Group 1 (Meats): 3 servings
Group 2 (Grains and Cereals): 1 serving
Group 3 (Vegetables and Fruits): 2 vegetable servings from List A
                                  or
                          1 serving from List A and
                          1 serving from List B
                          1 fruit serving
Group 4 (Milk): $1/_2$ serving*
Group 5 (Fats and Oils): 1 serving
Group 6 (Minimal Calories): Beverage and seasonings

• **BEDTIME SNACK**

Group 3 (Vegetables and Fruits): 1 vegetable serving from List A (optional)
                                  1 fruit serving
Group 4 (Milk): $1/_2$ serving*

  * You must have a total of 2 full Group 4 (Milk) servings every day. Divide them any way you
want, as long as they total 2 per day.

you will see the portion size that constitutes 1 serving. Simply select the food you want, in the number of servings and portion size specified. For avid calorie-counters, I've given the calories in a single portion in parentheses to the right of the food. The daily total of servings from all the groups will give you a weekly average of about 1,300 calories a day. For a sample menu, see pages 178–179.

Group 1: Meats

List A contains low-calorie meats and other high-protein foods; List B contains foods that are higher in fat and therefore in calories — so in many cases you get *twice* the amount of food in a single List A serving as you do for a single List B serving.

To reduce the amount of fat in your diet, you should try to eat at least 3 fish meals each week (preferably 5), and restrict your intake of beef, lamb, pork, and organ meats (liver, kidney, and heart) to no more than 3 meals per week.

Note that serving sizes and calories are for *cooked* portions, without bones, inedible parts, or any fat that you can cut away with a knife (including skin). No fat should be used in preparation. Pan juices, which can add many calories, are not included in the portions and calories given here.

LIST A

SERVING SIZE	FOOD	(CALORIES PER SERVING)
Fish		
2 oz.	Clams, canned or steamed	(60)
2 oz.	Cod or scrod steak or fillet	(60)
2 oz.	Crab	(60)
2 oz.	Flounder fillet	(60)
2 oz.	Haddock fillet	(60)
2 oz.	Halibut steak or fillet	(70)
2 oz.	Lobster	(60)
2 oz.	Mackerel (fresh)	(70)
2 oz.	Oysters, canned or steamed	(60)
2 oz.	Scallops	(60)
2 oz.	Shrimp	(60)
2 oz.	Snapper fillet, red or other	(70)

SERVING SIZE	FOOD	(CALORIES PER SERVING)
2 oz.	Sole fillet	(60)
2 oz.	Sturgeon	(70)
2 oz.	Swordfish	(70)
2 oz.	Trout (brook trout only)	(70)
¹/₂ cup	Tuna, canned in water, drained	(50)

Cheese

¹/₄ cup	Cottage cheese, dry curd	(40)
¹/₄ cup	Cottage cheese, 1–2% milk fat	(50)
¹/₄ cup	Cottage cheese, 4% milk fat	(60)
1 oz.	Ricotta cheese (part skim only) or plain farmer cheese	(45)

Legumes

3 oz.	Soybean curd (tofu), firm or soft type	(60)

List B

Meat

BEEF

1 oz.	Brisket	(65)
1 oz.	Chuck roast, lean	(60)
1 oz.	Flank steak	(55)
1 oz.	Foreshank	(55)
1 oz.	Ground round, lean	(60)
1 oz.	Heart	(55)
1 oz.	Liver	(65)
1 oz.	Round roast	(55)
1 oz.	Rump roast, lean	(60)
1 oz.	Sirloin steak, very lean, or other very lean steak	(65)
³/₄ oz. (ca. one half)	Frankfurter (all-beef — 1 average = ca. 1.6 oz.)	(70)

LAMB

1 oz.	Leg, lean	(60)
1 oz.	Loin, lean (chop, no bone)	(60)
1 oz.	Shoulder, lean (chop without bone; roast)	(60)

SERVING SIZE	FOOD	(CALORIES PER SERVING)
	PORK	
1 oz.	Boston butt roast	(70)
1 oz.	Chop, lean (broiled, no bone)	(75)
1½ slices as packaged, ca. 1 oz.	Ham, boiled or picnic	(70)
1 oz.	Ham roast, fresh or light-cured	(60)
1 oz.	Loin roast	(70)
	VEAL	
1 oz.	Chuck	(65)
1 oz.	Foreshank, stewed	(60)
1 oz.	Liver	(75)
1 oz.	Loin chop, medium fat	(65)
1 oz.	Round or rump; steak or cutlet	(60)
Poultry		
1 oz.	Chicken, dark or light, no skin	(55)
1 oz.	Chicken liver or heart	(50)
1 oz.	Turkey, dark or light, no skin	(55)
Fish		
¼ cup	Salmon, canned, drained	(55)
1 oz.	Salmon steak	(55)
3 medium	Sardines, drained of oil	(60)
¼ cup	Tuna, canned in oil, drained	(75)
Cheese*		
¾ oz.	Hard cheese: bleu, brick cheddar, Edam, Gouda, jack, mozzarella, Muenster, Port du Salut, provolone, Roquefort, Swiss	(80)
3 Tb.	Parmesan or Romano, grated	(65)
1 oz. (ca. 1½ slices, as packaged)	Processed American cheese	(100)
Eggs**		
1 medium	Egg (poached, boiled, or pan-cooked without fat)	(70)

SERVING SIZE	FOOD	(CALORIES PER SERVING)
Legumes		
¹/₄ cup	Dry beans or dry peas (i.e., black-eyed peas), cooked	(55)
¹/₄ cup	Lentils, cooked	(55)
¹/₄ cup	Kidney, white beans, or other canned beans, drained	(55)
1 Tb.	Peanut butter***	(100)

*Limit hard cheese to 4–6 meals per week.
**Limit eggs to 4–7 per week.
***Limit peanut butter to 1 serving per day.

Group 2: Grains and Cereals

BREAD (1 SLICE = CA. 1 OZ.)

SERVING SIZE	FOOD	(CALORIES PER SERVING)
¹/₂ small	Bagel	(70)
3 Tb.	Breadcrumbs	(60)
¹/₂ small	English muffin	(70)
¹/₂	Frankfurter roll	(70)
¹/₂	Hamburger bun	(60)
1 small	Pita bread or Mideastern sandwich pocket, white or whole wheat	(70)
1 average	Plain roll (cloverleaf, soft dinner roll)	(80)
1 oz.	Raisin bread, without sugar or icing	(75)
1 oz.	Rye or pumpernickel (soft type only)	(75)
1 small	Tortilla	(50)
1 oz.	White bread (including French, Italian types)	(75)
1 oz.	Whole-wheat bread	(75)

CRACKERS

3	Arrowroot	(60)
2 (2¹/₂" square)	Graham	(60)
¹/₂ (4" × 6")	Matzoh	(55)
3 (1¹/₂" × 3¹/₂")	Melba toast	(60)
20	Oyster	(60)
3 (2" × 3¹/₂")	Rye wafers	(60)
5	Saltines	(60)
4 (2¹/₂" square)	Soda	(60)

SERVING SIZE	FOOD	(CALORIES PER SERVING)

CEREALS

SERVING SIZE	FOOD	(CALORIES PER SERVING)
1 oz. (ca. $^2/_3$ cup)	Bran flakes	(90)
2 oz. cooked	Bulgar wheat	(110)
1 oz. ($^3/_4$–1 cup)	Cereal, ready to eat, unsweetened; i.e., corn flakes, shredded wheat, etc.	(110)
2 cups	Cereal, puffed, unfrosted	(110)
$^1/_2$ cup	Cereal, cooked; i.e., oatmeal, Cream of Wheat, etc.	(100)
$^1/_2$ cup	Cornmeal, cooked	(60)
2 Tb.	Cornstarch	(70)
$^1/_2$ cup	Egg noodles, cooked to tenderness	(100)
$2^1/_2$ Tb.	Flour	(50)
$^1/_2$ cup	Hominy grits, cooked	(120)
$^2/_3$ cup	Pasta, all types; i.e., macaroni, linguine, spaghetti, etc., cooked 14–20 minutes	(100)
3 cups	Popcorn, popped, no fat added	(75)
$^1/_2$ cup	Rice, brown, cooked	(100)
$^1/_4$ cup	Rice, Oriental, cooked	(110)
$^1/_2$ cup	Rice, white, cooked	(110)
$^1/_4$ cup (1 oz.)	Wheat germ	(110)

HIGH-STARCH VEGETABLES

Use these in your menu, if you wish, as a normal Group 2 serving. Note that they may not be eaten as a substitute for a Group 3 Vegetable serving.

SERVING SIZE	FOOD	(CALORIES PER SERVING)
$^1/_2$ cup	Corn	(80)
1 small	Corn on the cob	(70)
$^1/_2$ cup	Lima beans	(80)
3 oz. (1 small)	Potato, white (baked, boiled)	(70)
$^1/_2$ cup	Potato, mashed	(70)
$^1/_4$ cup	Yam or sweet potato	(60)

PREPARED BREADS

If you choose your Group 2 serving from these foods, eliminate one Group 5 (Fats and Oils) serving for that day.

SERVING SIZE	FOOD	(CALORIES PER SERVING)
1 (2″ diam.)	Biscuit	(100)
1 (2″ × 2″ × 1″ square)	Corn bread	(110)
1 ($1^1/_2$ oz.)	Bran muffin	(120)
1 ($1^1/_2$ oz.)	Corn muffin	(120)
1 (3″ diam.)	Plain muffin	(120)

Group 3: Vegetables and Fruits

Vegetables: List a (Low-Starch Vegetables)

SERVING SIZE	FOOD	(CALORIES PER SERVING)
$^1/_2$ cooked (leaves only)	Artichoke	(25)
8 oz. raw or 1 cup cooked	Asparagus	(30)
$^1/_2$ cup cooked	Beet greens	(15)
2 oz. raw or $^1/_2$ cup cooked	Bean sprouts	(20)
4 oz. raw or $^1/_2$ cup cooked	Broccoli	(20)
1 cup raw or $^1/_2$ cup cooked	Cabbage, red or white, shredded or chopped	(20)
1 6″ × 1″ raw or $^1/_2$ cup cooked	Carrot, trimmed	(25)
1 cup raw or $^3/_4$ cup cooked	Cauliflower buds	(20)
1 cup raw or cooked	Celery	(20)
$^1/_2$ cup cooked	Chard	(15)
3 cups raw	Chickory	(10)
3 cups raw	Chinese cabbage	(15)
$^1/_2$ cup cooked	Collard greens	(30)
1 cup raw	Cucumber	(20)
$^1/_2$ cup cooked	Eggplant	(20)
2 cups raw	Endive	(30)
2 cups raw	Escarole	(30)
1 cup raw or $^1/_2$ cup cooked	Green or bell pepper, diced or chopped	(20)
1 cup raw	Kale	(15)
3 cups raw	Lettuce: iceberg, Boston, romaine, etc.	(30)
1 cup raw or $^1/_2$ cup cooked	Mushrooms	(20)
$^1/_2$ cup cooked	Mustard greens	(25)
$^1/_2$ cup cooked	Okra	(25)
$^1/_2$ cup raw or cooked	Onion	(30)
2 (1″ × 1 $^3/_4$″ × 2″)	Pickles, dill, unsweetened	(30)
1 cup raw	Radishes	(20)
1 cup	Sauerkraut, drained	(30)
$^1/_2$ cup raw	Scallions (green onions, sliced)	(20)
2$^1/_2$ cups raw (trimmed) or 1 cup cooked	Spinach	(35)

SERVING SIZE	FOOD	(CALORIES PER SERVING)
¹/₂ cup raw (1¹/₂″ to 2″ pieces) or cooked	String beans, snap beans, green beans, or wax beans)	(20)
1¹/₂ cups raw or ¹/₂ cup cooked (just tender)	Summer squash (green, crookneck, zucchini, etc.)	(15)
1 small (ca. 4 to a pound) raw	Tomato	(20)
¹/₂ cup cooked	Tomatoes	(30)
³/₄ cup	Tomato juice	(35)
¹/₂ cup cooked	Turnip greens	(15)
¹/₂ cup cooked	Turnips, mashed	(25)
³/₄ cup	Vegetable juice cocktail	(35)
¹/₂ cup	Water chestnuts, canned, whole	(15)
3 cups raw	Watercress	(20)

VEGETABLES: LIST B (MEDIUM-STARCH VEGETABLES)

These vegetables are higher in starch than the preceding group. They must be cooked.

¹/₂ cup	Artichoke hearts, canned or frozen	(40)
¹/₂ cup	Beets, drained	(30)
¹/₂ cup (3–4 sprouts)	Brussels sprouts, cooked	(30)
¹/₂ cup	Parsnips, diced	(70)
¹/₂ cup	Peas, drained	(60–80)
¹/₂ cup	Pumpkin	(40)
¹/₂ cup	Rutabaga, diced	(30)
¹/₂ cup	Winter squash (yellow types)	(50)

FRUITS

1 small (2″ diam.)	Apple	(60)
¹/₃ cup	Apple juice	(60)
¹/₂ cup	Apple sauce, unsweetened	(50)
3 small	Apricots, fresh	(55)
4 halves	Apricots, dried	(50)
¹/₂ small	Banana	(40)
¹/₂ cup	Blackberries	(40)
¹/₂ cup	Blueberries	(45)
¹/₂ small	*Cantaloupe	(30)
10 large	Cherries	(55)
¹/₂ cup	Cider (nonalcoholic)	(60)
1 cup	*Cranberries, fresh, unsweetened	(50)

SERVING SIZE	FOOD	(CALORIES PER SERVING)
1 small (1½″ diam.)	Fig, fresh	(30)
1 (2″ × 1″)	Fig, dried	(60)
½ medium	*Grapefruit	(55)
½ cup	*Grapefruit juice, unsweetened	(55)
½ cup	Grapes	(60)
1 medium (ca. 3 to a pound)	Guava	(50)
½ cup or 2″ × 7″ wedge	Honeydew melon	(30)
½ cup (½ med.)	Mango, diced or sliced	(55)
1 small	*Orange	(55)
½ cup	*Orange juice	(55)
¾ cup	*Papaya, diced	(50)
1 medium (2″ diam., ca. 4 per pound)	Peach	(40)
1 small (ca. 4 per pound)	Pear, whole	(80)
½ cup	Pear, sliced, fresh	(50)
½ medium (ca. 2½″ diam.)	Persimmon, Japanese or Kaki	(40)
½ cup	*Pineapple:	
	Fresh, diced or sliced	(40)
	Canned in own juice, with 2 Tb. juice	(55)
⅓ cup	*Pineapple juice	(40)
2 medium (ca. 2″ diam. each)	Plums, fresh	(60)
4 medium (1 oz.)	Prunes, dried, soft, unsweetened	(65)
¼ cup	Prune juice	(50)
½ cup	Raspberries, fresh	(40)
2 Tb., loose	Raisins	(60)
1 cup	*Strawberries, fresh	(55)
1 large (ca. 4 to a pound)	*Tangerine	(40)
1 cup	Watermelon, diced	(45)

*Eat at least 1 serving of these fruits each day.

Group 4: Milk

SERVING SIZE	FOOD	(CALORIES PER SERVING)
1 cup	Buttermilk, cultured:	
	From skim milk	(75)
	Less than 1% fat	(90)
	1% fat	(100)

SERVING SIZE	FOOD	(CALORIES PER SERVING)
½ cup	Canned evaporated skim milk, before adding water	(100)
½ cup	Canned evaporated whole milk, before adding water	(170)
½ cup	*Ice cream, plain only	(150)
⅓ cup dry	Powdered nonfat dry milk, before adding liquid	(100)
1 cup	Skim milk:	(90)
	Nonfat (skimmed)	
	Low-fat (partially skimmed)	(145)
1 cup	Whole milk	(160)
⅔ cup	Yogurt made from skim milk (low-fat, plain only)	(100)

*Do not eat ice cream more than once a week. The brand and flavor must not contain more than 150 calories per half cup.

Group 5: Fats and Oils

SERVING SIZE	FOOD	(CALORIES PER SERVING)
⅛ (4″ diam.)	Avocado	(45)
1 strip, thin	*Bacon, crisp, drained	(35)
1 tsp.	*Butter	(35)
1 Tb.	*Cream, heavy	(50)
2 Tb.	*Cream, light	(60)
2 Tb.	*Cream, sour	(60)
1 Tb.	*Cream cheese	(60)
1 tsp.	*Lard or meat drippings	(35)
1 tsp.	Margarine	(35)
2 tsp.	Margarine, reduced-calorie	(35)
1 tsp.	Mayonnaise	(35)
2 tsp.	Mayonnaise, reduced-calorie	(35)
6 small	Nuts, mixed (choose dry-roasted if possible)	(45)
1 tsp.	Oil (corn, cottonseed, olive, peanut, safflower, soybean, sunflower)	(45)
5 small	Olives, green or smooth black	(30)
1 Tb.	Reduced-calorie or low-calorie condiments, jellies, salad dressings, and syrups that contain *not more than 30 calories per tablespoon* (as stated on product's label)	(30)
2 tsp.	Salad dressing, French (orange type)	(35)

SERVING SIZE	FOOD	(CALORIES PER SERVING)
1½ tsp. (½ Tb.)	Salad dressing: Italian, bleu cheese, or mayonnaise type	(40)
¼" cube	*Salt pork	(40)

*These contain saturated fats.

Group 6: Minimal Calories—Herbs, Spices, and Beverages

These foods are so low in calories in the amounts in which they are normally used that you do not need to measure them.

Broth: beef, chicken, or onion broth, fat-free only, made from cubes or individual packets*
Celery salt
Chili powder
Coffee, regular or decaffeinated
Garlic
Gelatin, unsweetened
Ground herbs; i.e., basil, marjoram, dill, tarragon, savory, etc.
Ground spices; i.e., cinnamon, nutmeg, cloves, curry, etc.
Herbal teas (contain no caffeine)
Horseradish, white or red
Lemon juice and lemon peel (as flavoring only)
Lime juice and lime peel (as flavoring only)

Mint
Mustard, prepared or dry
Onion flakes
Onion salt or powder
Paprika
Pepper, black or red
Salt
Seltzer water or soda water
Soft drinks, low-calorie
Soy sauce
Steak sauce
Tabasco sauce
Vanilla
Vinegar: white; cider; red wine or white wine vinegar
Worcestershire sauce

*These have a high salt content

SOME RULES TO FOLLOW

• Do not add or omit any servings. Never skip a meal, and never "carry over" a serving to the next day. If you skip a serving on Monday, you may *not* make up for it by eating an additional serving on Tuesday.
• Choose only the foods specified in the Getting Thin Diet as long as you are trying to lose weight.
• You may divide and combine portions as you like, as long as they add up to the serving specified for that meal, no more and no less. For instance, instead of eating one whole fruit for dessert at dinner, you may

want to combine a half-serving of one fruit with a half-serving of another as a fruit compote.

- Make sure you choose a variety of foods from each food group. Don't eat the same thing from each group day after day. As you learned in Chapter 11, nearly all foods provide a combination of nutrients. Eating a variety of foods will ensure your getting adequate amounts of each one.
- Finally, invest in a good, accurate kitchen scale. It should be easy to read, and able to weigh foods up to one pound or more. It should also have a container that will hold soft or runny foods, and be easy to clean. When preparing meals, *weigh and measure everything scrupulously as long as you are trying to lose weight.* (Remember to allow for the weight of the container.)

SOME THINGS TO AVOID

I don't want you to think of the Getting Thin Diet in terms of "don'ts." This is an abundant and varied eating plan with lots of room for freedom of choice. There are, however, a few sensible precautions you must take to keep your calories at or under the 1,300 daily mark and get adequate nutrition.

- Avoid prepared foods, such as soups, or frozen precooked meals, while you are trying to lose weight. If you must eat prepared foods — which are often made with sugar or fats that add hidden calories — try to determine the calorie content first by looking on the package label or checking a brand-name calorie counter.
- Don't cook with fats. Forget fried foods, and don't add butter, margarine, cooking oil, or animal fat in preparing food. Bake, stew, or broil your meats. If you're in the habit of using the juices that cook out of animal products and using them as gravy, break it. Natural juices are almost entirely fat.
- Fat is concentrated in the skins of all animals, including fish and poultry. Always remove skins before eating these foods.
- Eliminate sugar and sugary sweets — jams, jellies, candy, syrups, and pastries. Use the natural sweetness of fruits to help pacify your sweet tooth, as well as noncaloric sugar substitutes.
- Avoid alcoholic beverages. You can drink later, when you are maintaining your weight, but not while you're losing weight. Alcohol is a specific chemical not classifiable as carbohydrate, protein, or fat, but it does have calories — seven per gram. It is a dense source of otherwise worthless

A One-Day Sample Menu from the Getting Thin Diet

MEAL	GROUP	SERVINGS	FOODS
• BREAKFAST	1	1	3/4 oz. melted cheddar cheese
	2	1	1/2 small English muffin
	3	1 Fruit	1/2 cup orange juice
	4	1/2	1/2 cup skim milk
	5	1	1 slice crisp bacon
	6		Coffee (with skim milk, you have *café au lait*)
• MIDMORNING SNACK	4	1/2	1/3 cup yogurt, blended with
	6	(optional)	1 cup chicken broth, made from cube and flavored with dill
• LUNCH	1	2	1 1/2 slices boiled ham and 3/4 oz. Swiss cheese with mustard
	2	2	2 slices rye bread
	3	1 List A Veg.	2 cups salad made with romaine lettuce, sliced mushrooms, cucumber, scallions, radishes
	5	1	1/2 Tb. Italian salad dressing
	6		Coffee, tea, seltzer, or low-cal. soft drink
• AFTERNOON SNACK	3	1 List A Veg. (optional)	1 6" raw shredded carrot, mixed with
	3	1 Fruit	1/4 cup chopped pineapple and 1 Tb. raisins, flavored with

calories and it loosens your inhibitions and thus undermines your will power. However, if you feel that in certain situations you *must* have a drink, choose a small glass of dry wine.

- Choose whole-wheat and whole-grain foods over white breads, pastas, and other foods made with refined or polished flour. Twenty-one known nutrients are removed from this flour in the refining process, and only

MEAL	GROUP	SERVINGS	FOODS
	6	(optional)	Dash of nutmeg or cinnamon Coffee, tea, seltzer, or low-cal. soft drink
• DINNER	1	3	6 oz. broiled swordfish steak, basted with soy sauce and fresh lemon, *or* 3 oz. broiled chicken breast (baste with skim milk; remove skin before eating)
	2	1	1 small baked potato with
	5	1	2 Tb. sour cream
	3	2 List A Vegs. or 1 from List A and 1 from List B	$^1/_2$ artichoke, cooked (List A) *and* $^1/_2$ cup green beans, cooked (List A) *or* $^1/_2$ cup peas (List B)
	3	1 Fruit	1 cup fresh strawberries, flavored with
	4	$^1/_2$	$^1/_4$ cup evaporated skim milk, $^1/_2$ tsp. vanilla, and
	6		Pinch of cinnamon
	6		Coffee (decaffeinated) or herbal tea
• BEDTIME SNACK	3	1 Fruit	$^1/_2$ small banana, blended with
	4	$^1/_2$	$^1/_2$ cup skim milk and
	6		$^1/_4$ tsp. vanilla and a pinch of freshly grated nutmeg

five are replaced later. The polished flour products may be no more fattening than their unrefined counterparts, but they give you less nutrition per calorie.
• Try to use as many high-fiber grain and cereal products as possible. For instance, eat brown rice rather than white rice. Cutting down on calories can lead to constipation unless you eat a lot of fiber.

Is it Safe to Use Saccharin?

Saccharin is a nonnutritive chemical sweetener that many people use in place of sugar. Since 1970, scientists in the United States and Canada have been conducting tests to see if any link can be established between this artificial sweetener and cancer in humans.

The evidence to suggest a link between saccharin and cancer in humans is so slight as to be insignificant. In 1977, a Canadian study showed that pregnant guinea pigs who were given saccharin in amounts that would be equivalent to that found in 800 to 1,300 soft drinks a day did produce offspring with bladder cancer. Studies conducted since then with human subjects have failed to demonstrate any association between cancer of the bladder, or any other cancer, and taking saccharin.

Obviously, few of you are going to ingest saccharin in amounts coming anywhere near the equivalent of 800 sugar-free soft drinks a day. If you feel that you cannot survive a diet without the use of an artificial sweetener, I would not prohibit you from drinking sugar-free soft drinks or using saccharin to flavor desserts. But because the evidence is not conclusive one way or another, I suggest you limit the use of saccharin as much as possible, especially if you are uneasy about the risk, however slight. Better yet, use your new, healthier way of eating on the Getting Thin Diet to help yourself break the sweet-tooth habit, and learn to enjoy the clean taste of seltzer water with a twist of lemon or the naturally sweet taste of fresh fruits.

- Reduced-calorie breads are fine, but don't use thin-sliced breads. One slice should weigh one ounce.
- Most popular cereal brands are loaded with sugar. Read labels carefully before you buy, and avoid the cereals with high sugar content. Instead, pick one of the many tasty cereals that are rich in fiber but have little or no sugar.
- Drink skim milk instead of whole or "low-fat" milk. Some producers of "low-fat" skim milk take out 1 or 2 percent of the milk fat only to replace it with high-protein milk solids. The skim milk may taste better this way, but it has the same number of calories as whole milk. Buy milk that is labeled zero percent fat. (For a richer flavor, try adding $1/4$ teaspoon vanilla to 1 cup of skim milk.)
- Look for cheese that are made from skim or part-skim milk, and choose low-fat yogurts. The yogurts should be fruit-free as well as low-fat. Most manufacturers add sugar to yogurt along with the fruit, and this increases the calorie content quite a bit. Plain yogurt has about 150 calories per cup, while fruited yogurt may have as many as 250 — as much as ice cream.

WHAT TO EXPECT

As you learned earlier in this chapter, you should lose about 2 pounds of fat a week on the Getting Thin Diet if you exercise. But you may not always lose the same amount of *weight*. There are several reasons why.

Early Water Loss

I mentioned earlier that you experienced dieters may be used to losing as much as 6 or 7 pounds in your first week of dieting, much of it water. Water loss amounting to several pounds is not unusual in the first few days of a low-carbohydrate diet.

As you already know, a diet very low in carbohydrates can deplete the sugar stored in your liver in about twelve hours. Each gram of lost sugar carries with it three grams of water. A low-carbohydrate diet causes ketones to build up in your bloodstream. They act on your kidneys to make you urinate more and lose fluid. This initial water loss will not occur on the Getting Thin Diet because the diet is not low in carbohydrates.

Nevertheless, there probably will be some changes in your water-loss pattern during the diet. You probably will urinate a little more frequently. This will indicate that your stored fat is breaking down and being lost. As you learned in Chapter 3, water is one of the breakdown products of fat metabolism.

The First Week

Most of you will find that you lose more weight during the first week of your diet than at any other stage. The loss may be as much as 4 or 5 pounds in the first week, especially if you are very overweight when you start to diet.

This big initial loss is *not* an excessive loss of water, but a true loss of fat.

Size plays a large part in determining your calorie needs, as you will discover in Chapter 15. The more pounds you're carrying, the bigger the deficit you're creating when you start to diet. In other words, the more you have to lose, the more quickly you'll be able to lose in the early days of your diet. This should be an encouraging thought.

Delayed Water Loss

A few of you may find that you don't lose any weight at all for the first two or three weeks of your diet, even though you follow the diet carefully and exercise as well.

Don't be discouraged. Even if you aren't losing pounds, you *are* losing fat.

Science can't tell us why, but people's patterns of water loss vary widely. If you don't lose pounds in your first two or three weeks of dieting, it is only because you are retaining water.

Anywhere between the diet's tenth and twenty-fifth day, you probably will begin urinating profusely. A day or two of high-volume urination will leave you with the weight loss you might have expected had you been losing gradually all along.

Leveling Off and Plateauing

By the third week of the diet, both the big early losers and the big late losers should have leveled off. From here on, you can expect to lose a steady 2 pounds or so each week — until you near your ideal weight.

As you get closer to your goal, weight loss will come harder. You will have reached the "plateau" bemoaned by many dieters. The source of your problem is your diminished calorie needs. Lost pounds have made your body smaller, and even your firmed-up muscles with their new-found calorie-burning capacity can't create a calorie demand to make up for the lost burden. It may take two weeks or so for you to create a large enough calorie deficit to cause the loss of a single pound.

Persevere. You should be well into the swing of your new diet and exercise habits by now, so dieting should seem easier and more natural. Besides, you should be delighted to be so near your goal.

Weighing In

While you're on your diet, weigh yourself no more than once a week. Weighing more often can be disappointing, and it certainly is misleading. There are too many variables that can change your weight from day to day without reflecting any true loss or gain of fat. These variables include:

- The water retention we just talked about, along with the special water retention problems of women. As you know, water retention caused by female hormones can amount to up to 5 pounds of fluid weight gain in some women every month.
- Dehydration. You can sweat off as many as 5 pounds in a hard workout. Don't deceive yourself. The water weight will return once you eat or drink.
- Elimination. Either moving your bowels or excreting a mere pint of urine can make you a pound lighter temporarily.
- The time of day. You don't weigh the same before you eat as you do after, a fact that can confuse you if you try to weigh yourself daily at different times.

Inches before Pounds

There is also the matter of muscles to consider. If you are dieting and exercising properly, you are building up and firming your muscles while you lose fat. Muscles weigh more than fat. So it's possible that your weight can stabilize, or even increase slightly, at the same time you're losing fat.

For this reason, the scale is not your most reliable indicator of progress. Turn instead to the tape measure. Take a weekly reading of your waist, hips, and thighs. As long as they are getting smaller you are losing fat, no matter what the scale says.

When You Reach Your Goal

You've made it! You've lost every last pound and inch you wanted to lose!

What do you do now?

I have two recommendations:

First, cheat. Invite the neighbors in, open a bottle of fattening champagne, and help them drink it. Your feat deserves a celebration.

Second, quit cheating. Get back down to the business of pursuing your lifetime commitment to slenderness and health. Never forget that your diet was not a temporary episode, but the foundation for eating habits that are supposed to last forever.

You must now learn to eat so that your calorie needs and your calorie intake balance. This means that you can eat more than the 1,300 calories a day you ate on the Getting Thin Diet.

But how much more?

Individuals vary so much that there's really no accurate scientific formula that will tell you this in advance. Roughly speaking, a woman of average height between the ages of twenty and fifty-five, who leads a moderately active life — as I define that in Chapter 15 — will probably need anywhere from 1,800 TO 2,100 calories a day to maintain her weight at a steady level. A male of the same description might need anywhere from 2,100 to 2,500.

The way to find out what's right for you — your maintenance calorie level — is to add calories the way you took off pounds: *slowly and gradually*. This is how the Staying Thin Food Plan works.

THE STAYING THIN FOOD PLAN

Like the Getting Thin Diet itself, the principle here is simple. Using the chart on page 185, just add the number of servings indicated for each food group to the basic 1,300–calorie diet in order to raise your daily calorie intake gradually to your maintenance level.

Start by raising your calorie intake to 1,400 a day. If you look at the "1,400" column of the chart, you will see that this means adding on *one* serving from the Grains and Cereals list and *one* serving from the Fruits list. Adding this much to the Getting Thin Diet gives you 1,400 calories a day. You should maintain this level for two weeks.

Then add another 100 calories. If you look at the "1,500" column, you will see the total number of servings that should be added to the basic 1,300–calorie plan to give you about 1,500 calories a day: *one* serving from the Meats Group, *one* from Grains and Cereals, *one* from Fruits, and *one* Fat serving.

Important note: the numbers in each column mean that this is what you add on to the Getting Thin 1,300–Calorie Diet. *Do not add on to the previous column*. Thus: on the Getting Thin Diet you have 4 fruits a day. At 1,500, you have one more, or 5; at 2,100, two more, or 6; at 2,600, three more, or 7 fruits a day, total.

Keep on adding 100 calories a week every two weeks, and weigh yourself once a week. Eventually, depending on your sex, age, and level of activity, you will find that you are no longer losing, and that you have even gained back one or two pounds. This slight fluctuation shows that you have reached the upper limit of your maintenance calorie level.

The Staying Thin Food Plan

(Figures represent the number of servings to add to the basic 1,300-calorie diet to increase calories by 100 a day.)

THE CALORIE LEVEL YOU WANT TO REACH

FOOD GROUPS	1400	1500	1600	1700	1800	1900	2000	2100	2200	2300	2400	2500	2600	2700	2800
GROUP 1: Meats	1	1	1	1	1	1½	2½	3	3	3	4	4	5	5	5
GROUP 2: Grains and Cereals	1	1	2	2	2	3	3½	3½	5	6	6	6	6	7	7½
GROUP 3: Vegetables					2	2	2	2	2	2	2	2	2	2	2
Fruits	1				1	1	1	2	2	2	2	2	3	3	3
GROUP 4: Milk				½	½	½	½	½	½	½	½	1	1	1½	2
GROUP 5: Fats and Oils	1	1	1	1	1	1	1	2	2	3	3	4	4	4	5

Now, drop 100 calories from your daily intake — that is, go back one column — and weigh yourself weekly for a month to see if your weight stabilizes. This is the calorie level at which you can expect to maintain your weight, and your glorious new figure, as long as you also maintain your present level of activity.

But remember, *you must maintain your new habits along with that calorie level.* Sticking to an exercise program will allow you to keep your eating habits and your weight on an even keel. And though you can eat more, you should not eat differently. A thin wedge of pie or a small piece of cake once in a while won't hurt. But don't confuse a minor fling with lapsing back into the old eating habits that helped make you fat. *Weigh once a week*, and take your measurements once a week. The moment you find yourself creeping over the two or three pounds you started to gain back at maintenance level, nip the slippage in the bud by returning to the basic Getting Thin Diet.

You have, in advance, my hearty congratulations on your successful diet. But don't forget that dieting is only one-third the battle. Changing your ways of dealing with the problems food poses and learning to exercise properly are also essential, and you're about to learn a lot more about these two vital elements.

14.

BEHAVIOR MODIFICATION: HOW TO EAT

How many chronic dieters have noticed this ironic problem: when you diet, all you can think about is food. You fantasize about the pizzas you'll gorge on, the milk shakes you'll guzzle, as soon as you get thin. You may be depriving your body to the point of misery, but your mind is still thinking fat.

Clearly, you're setting yourself up to yo-yo. You may be doing without your favorite foods, but you're not attacking your craving for them. You may be losing weight, but you're not dealing with the habits that made you fat in the first place. You're just holding them temporarily in check.

Along with exercise, the most important factor in permanent weight control is to change the relationship between you and food. You have to alter your basic attitudes toward eating.

This is easier said than done, but it's by no means impossible. A good method for doing it is through a technique called *behavior modification*.

HOW IT STARTED

Obesity can be almost as frustrating for experts who treat it as for people who suffer from it.

One expert who can testify to this is Albert J. Stunkard. You met Dr. Stunkard in Chapter 10 as the author of the famous Manhattan Study on obesity and socioeconomic class. He has headed the departments of psychiatry at the medical schools of both Stanford and the University of Pennsylvania, and he's one of the world's leading authorities on fat. Yet there was a point in his career when he was almost convinced that no truly effective treatment for obesity existed.

He found that of patients being treated by doctors for overweight, no more than 25 percent lost as much as 20 pounds. Only 5 percent lost as much as 40 pounds. These depressing statistics held, no matter what kind of treatment was used. Intense psychotherapy could help some people control their weight permanently, but only at an exorbitant cost in years, effort, and dollars. Obviously, it was no answer to changing eating habits for the vast majority of fat people.

The Stuart Findings

Then, several years ago, Dr. Stunkard ran across a short article in an obscure technical journal. It was called "Behavioral Control of Overeating." Its author was Richard Stuart, then a professor of social work at the University of Michigan.

The article detailed the histories of eight patients over the course of one year of medical treatment for obesity designed to change their approach to food and eating. Of these patients, not one fourth, but *all*, lost more than 20 pounds. Not 5 percent, but *half*, lost more than 40 pounds.

Dr. Stunkard launched an experiment to see if he could duplicate this staggering success by using Stuart's techniques. He set up two groups of patients. One was treated with conventional methods of diet and therapy, the other with behavior modification. The results:

- In the first group, 24 percent lost 20 pounds or more, and no one lost as much as 40 pounds. In the behavior therapy group, 53 percent lost more than 20 pounds, and 13 percent lost more than 40 pounds.
- None of the first group lost even as much as 30 pounds, but 33 percent of the behavior modification group did.
- None of the behavior therapy patients dropped out of treatment. Dropout rates with conventional treatment generally range from 20 to 80 percent.
- None of the behavior modification group reported any bad side effects whatever from the treatment.
- After one year, all the patients who had lost more than 20 pounds with behavior modification had maintained the loss. Three of them had lost another 20 pounds each. One patient who had lost 40 pounds during treatment had lost more than 100 pounds by the end of the year of follow-up.

The success of Stuart, Stunkard, and other pioneers in behavior modification has firmly established the technique as a valuable and effective aid in long-term weight control.

HOW IT WORKS

Behavior modification rests on the externality theory I talked about in Chapter 7. It seems that thin people eat when their bodies tell them they're hungry. In other words, they respond to internal cues. Fat people, on the other hand, appear to eat in response to cues from their environment. They may respond more to the taste, smell, and general sensual appeal of food. And, the theory goes, they are more inclined to eat in reaction to some emotional state.

Behavior modification is based on the idea that if you can find out what external cues make you eat, you can change your eating habits.

Here are the four main components of behavior modification:
- Find out what external cues make you eat.
- Control those cues.
- Control the act of eating.
- Reward your successes in mastering your eating behavior.

Finding the Cues

Your first step in changing bad eating habits is to pinpoint exactly what those habits are.

Do you stuff the car's glove compartment with candy bars so you can eat while you drive? Do you down six beers while watching a football game on television? Do you sample food all day long while you cook for your family? When grocery shopping, do you impulsively pick up potato chips or cookies that weren't on your shopping list?

Do you eat until you're full, or until the food runs out? Do you eat to celebrate? To mourn? Do you eat when you're happy, bored, insecure, depressed, angry, or nervous?

The questions may seem simple. But the fact is, most overeaters are unaware of the cues that make them overeat — and therefore are powerless to control them.

The way to discover these cues is to keep a detailed diary of eating. It should be small enough to carry around with you at all times — I suggest a small spiral notebook. Every scrap of food you eat goes into the diary. The only exceptions are water and other noncaloric fluids. And you have to keep track of more than just food. You must record:
- When you eat
- Where and with whom you eat

- What prompts you to eat
- What mood you're in
- How hungry you are
- What else you may be doing while you eat
- How much you eat
- How many calories you take in.

Keep this diary as long as you are trying to lose weight. Even after only a week or two, a pattern will emerge that will tell you a surprising number of things about yourself and your eating habits. By studying this pattern and coming to understand it better, you will know much more about what foods, moods, circumstances, and other external cues tend to trigger a craving for food even when you are not actually hungry. You will be able to anticipate when you may want to overeat, and nip binges in the bud. (In fact, you will probably find that just writing down your feelings and being more aware of them will take the edge off your craving for food.)

Keeping the diary is usually laborious, boring, unsettling — and very effective. It brings you face to face with your bad habits, and that kind of confrontation isn't very pleasant. It is, however, very necessary. You must know the enemy to defeat him.

If you don't want to construct your own diary, a good ready-made one is available. It's a spiral notebook called *The Eat & Run Calendar*, by Jan Ferris Koltun (Holt, Rinehart and Winston, $8.70). The calendar is updated every year. Along with log pages, it contains some helpful tips on behavior and some cartoons to amuse you.

Changing the Cues

You may find from keeping your diary that you eat for every reason under the sun except the right one — being hungry. So you set about training yourself to listen to your body instead of your environment.

If you find that you eat while driving, make sure you keep no food in the car. If you eat while watching TV, replace the habit with a hobby like knitting or sketching that will occupy your mind and hands. Better yet, find a form of exercise that you can do in front of the television. Ride a stationary bicycle, or work out on a mini-trampoline. If you can substitute exercise for eating, you're got it made.

Shop for food only when you're full. That way, fattening food won't seem so alluring. If you're a chronic snacker, budget your daily calorie intake into a number of small meals. Carry low-calorie snacks like raw vegetables along with you to ward off the urge to stop by the candy-vending machine or wolf down two doughnuts on your morning coffee break.

If leaving leftovers makes you feel guilty, find or invent some low-calorie recipes for them, and set aside a day or two each week for meals made only of leftovers.

If you eat when you're depressed, try turning to a friend for comfort instead of the refrigerator. Learn to talk about your problems.

There's a list of hints later in the chapter to help you modify your eating behavior. Take careful note of the suggestions, and feel free to add ideas of your own that may suit your special case.

Controlling the Act of Eating

Many fat people are gobblers. They may be so intent on the taste of food that they eat it ravenously, overloading before their bodies have a chance to signal a halt.

If this is your problem, your main task is to learn to eat slowly. Remember, it takes about twenty minutes for most people to begin to feel full after eating. Give your food time to satisfy you, and you'll want less and eat less.

Along with timing, eating rituals are important. We humans tend to construct routines around the act of eating, so that eating becomes linked in our minds to certain activities or locations. For instance, we may become accustomed to eating while we read a newspaper, or eating anytime we enter the kitchen. After a while, picking up a newspaper or walking into the kitchen becomes a cue to eat.

The best way to break this stimulus-response linkage is to make eating a separate act in and of itself, unrelated to any other pursuit. Make eating a ritual of its own. Limit the locations where you allow yourself to eat. Don't read, talk on the telephone, or watch television while you eat. Devote your full attention to your food.

Rewards

Congratulate yourself for changing your ways by giving yourself little rewards.

This will work best if the rewards are reasonable and frequent. Don't promise yourself a Rolls-Royce for losing 60 pounds. Instead, treat yourself to a new scarf or tie if you've spent a week substituting carrot sticks for pastries as snacks. Or go out to a movie as a reward for having exercised for thirty minutes three times in one week.

Rewards are essential in retraining your habits. They reinforce and underscore your victories. They also help you associate pleasure with proper eating. This can help replace the pleasure you once found in overeating.

TIPS FOR RESHAPING YOUR EATING HABITS

Behavior modification has been so successful that many diet books, good and bad, devote some space to the subject. There are even a number of books that deal only with the technique itself. If you collected all the variations on the theme, your list of behavior tips would be so long that your life would be unmanageably complicated.

To keep matters as simple and pleasant as possible, I offer what I consider to be the sanest and most effective suggestions.

While Shopping

The American supermarket is an invitation to overweight. Regard it as the mine field that it is, and be sure to:
- Shop only after a satisfying meal. Being full helps you resist temptation.
- *Never* go marketing without a grocery list. Having a list will get you through the store as fast as possible and discourage impulse buying of fattening foods.
- Make another list — this one of fattening foods that tend to make you go off your diet. Put them on the list. Then make it a point to *avoid* these foods when you shop — stay away from the aisles where they are located. If you don't see them, you won't buy them to take home. If they're not around the house, you won't eat them.
- Be aware of foods that you can use as substitutes for more fattening foods that you find tempting. For instance, if you're inclined to buy steak to prepare as a dinner entrée, list and buy a broiling chicken instead.
- If you have to buy fattening foods for nondieters at home, choose varieties that you yourself don't particularly like. For instance, if chocolate ice cream is your favorite, leave it alone and buy pistachio for the kids.
- Read labels. The plots may be dull, but the information is vital. There's

no other way to be sure how much sugar you're buying in your morning cereal, or how much fat is tucked away in a TV dinner or frozen entrée. If a particular packaged food is not properly labeled, pass it up.

- Avoid hidden fats. The fat on a cut of meat is easy to spot. The fat in an avocado isn't. Get to know the less obvious high-fat foods, and find substitutes for them or do without them altogether. Look for low-fat and part-skim cheeses, no-fat milk, tuna fish packed in water instead of oil. Avoid processed meats. Most of them are loaded with fat.

At Home and Work

- Enlist your family, friends, and workmates in the cause. Let them know you're cutting down. Tell them they can be kindest by being stingy with offers of second helpings and fattening treats.
- Do you have a friend who is also trying to lose weight? Try a partnership approach to dieting, exercise, and moral support. Perhaps you could shop together or join the same aerobics dance class. Arrange to call the friend when you need help and encouragement in resisting the craving for food. Both of you may find that understanding is a good appetite suppressant.
- Be mindful of temptation when you arrange your refrigerator and kitchen cabinets. In deference to members of the household who may not be weight-conscious, you may have to keep some fattening items about. But you needn't put them in places where they pop immediately into view as soon as you open the pantry or refrigerator door.
- Don't do your socializing, television watching, reading, needlework, carpentry, or whatever in the kitchen. The kitchen should be the place for keeping food, preparing meals, and, in some households, eating meals. Being there for any other reason may tempt you to overeat.
- Devote your leisure time to food-free activities. Exercise is the best pursuit of all. Failing that, however, take up some activity to substitute for eating that you habitually associate with certain cues. Knit, don't eat, while you watch TV.
- If coffee breaks at work mean more than coffee, skip them. Take a brisk walk instead. Or, boss permitting, spend a pleasant few minutes chatting with a friend on the phone.
- Forget the two-martini business lunch, and avoid alcohol. You can be just as sociable over a glass of mineral water with a lime twist. You can be more sociable still with a quick noontime game of racquetball. Alcohol is a dense, nonnutritious source of calories. It's an appetite stimulant. And it sabotages your willpower by easing your inhibitions.
- Bring your lunch to work whenever possible instead of going out to a

restaurant. Restaurants are in the business of serving tasty foods, and tasty food is usually high in fat. You're in the business of changing your habits. You'll have more control if you prepare your own food instead of leaving if up to a chef.

When You Eat Out

Man is a social being, and none of us lives in a vacuum. Eating out is a pleasant and sometimes necessary social activity, and it's pointless to try to avoid it altogether. But here are some ways to minimize the calorie costs of restaurant meals:

- Stick to mineral water instead of alcohol during premeal cocktails. Alcohol is rarely "unavoidable." But if you feel that you cannot refuse a drink, make it one small glass of dry wine and nurse it through the meal — if possible, accompany it with a mineral-water chaser.
- Leave the rolls and butter to your companions. One hard roll with butter can add 300 calories to your meal.
- Order a big salad before the main course, and dress it with lemon or with a small lacing of oil and vinegar. This will help curb your appetite for the balance of the meal.
- Choose poultry or fish as an entrée rather than meat. Request that your selection be prepared without butter or cooking oil. It may, for instance, be broiled "dry" with only lemon juice. Never be afraid to send a dish back if it doesn't conform to your specifications.
- If you can't avoid ordering a fattening entrée, eat only a half portion. Scrape off the sauce first.
- If you want dessert, forget the éclairs and baked Alaska and order fruit instead. Or you may want to adopt the European custom of finishing a meal, instead of starting one, with a salad. It refreshes your palate and leaves you feeling light, not sugary and sodden.

As a Dinner Guest in Someone's Home

Dining out in friends' homes is a little trickier than dining out in a restaurant. You have to be careful not to let your weight-loss program interfere with your good manners, or vice versa. Here are some ways to minimize potential problems:

- Let your host or hostess know well in advance that you're dieting. If he or she offers to prepare some low-calorie specialties, accept with thanks. If not, you're at least prepared your excuse for eating only limited portions. Not mentioning your diet will only increase the chance that you'll eat too much, or that you'll offend someone by neglecting an elaborate, high-calorie dinner.

- If you suspect a rich meal has been planned, gird yourself ahead of time to resist temptation. Have a substantial but low-calorie snack before leaving home to blunt your appetite for the fattening dinner ahead.
Say no, thank you to the predinner hors d'oeuvres.
- Drink mineral water or low-calorie soft drinks instead of a cocktail. Avoid alcohol before dinner — it will just make eating at dinner harder to control. If you cannot politely say no to wine with dinner, nurse it slowly and drink no more than a small glass.

General Guidelines for Meals

- Eat slowly. This is the most important mealtime tip of all, so do whatever it takes to make it work. Put less food on your fork or spoon. Try to chew each bite twenty times before you swallow. If you have to, count the number of bites you take. Put down your fork or spoon between every bite. All this may be tedious, but you'll soon learn to slow down, and eating slowly will begin to seem natural and make food taste better. Remember the twenty-minute rule for feeling full. If you feel like having seconds, hold off the urge for at least twenty minutes. By that time, it should be controllable.
- Eat three meals a day, as well as three snacks of the type I recommend in the Getting Thin Diet in Chapter 13. Keep them small, but never skip them. Contradictory as it may sound, it's important that when dieting you never let yourself get hungry. Skipping a meal puts you at risk of overeating at the next meal. And as you know, controlled frequent eating encourages the proper functioning of some metabolic factors, notably insulin response and brown-fat activity.
- When you eat, do nothing else — no television, no reading, no phone calls or paper work. Concentrate on the taste, smells, appearance, and texture of your food. You'll savor it more, and less will seem like more. This method will also help eliminate the mental links that make certain activities prompt you to eat.
- Set aside one place in your home for eating — preferably the kitchen or dining-room table — and eat there and nowhere else. This should apply to everything you eat, snacks as well as meals. By doing this, you'll cut down on the number of places you associate with food. You'll also make yourself more aware of what and when you eat.
- Before you eat so much as a celery stalk, set out a place mat and a complete dining service at your usual eating spot. Again, this will help you assess your food intake by making you pay more attention to it. It

may also make eating such a chore that you won't bother with it. Of course, this applies only to food you eat at home, not to the permitted low-calorie snacks on the Diet, which you take with you to work or elsewhere to smother temptation during the day.

- Drink at least one glass of water before meals and another glass with the meal. You'll feel fuller.
- Serve meals in portions set out in the kitchen before you sit down to eat. Decide before you start that you're going to eat what's on your plate and no more. Never have "family-style" meals with platters of food laid out on the table. This arrangement encourages you to take second helpings.
- Serve yourself small portions on small plates. The smaller portions will look bigger this way. You'll soon find that the portions that once looked skimpy to you are perfectly adequate to fill you up.
- Start the meal with something hot. Low-calorie hot soups are ideal. Hot foods slow down your eating and give you more time to feel full.
- Eat the foods you like best first. You'll feel more satisfied and more inclined to quit once you've moved on to the less tasty foods.
- If possible, have someone else in the household clear the table and put away the leftovers. You'll be less likely to keep munching after the meal is finished.
- If you can't bring yourself to throw food away but don't like to eat leftovers later, give them to a pet. If you don't have one, offer the leftovers to your neighbors for their cat or dog — or rabbit or gerbil or wildebeest. Just make sure the disposal unit you use is not your own body.

LOW CALORIES AND HIGH MORALE

It sometimes seems that the weight-watcher's life is fraught with pitfalls. Your appetite and your environment seem to conspire to make you overeat. Making the transition from bad habits to a healthier lifestyle may be very trying emotionally.

But it's important to hold on to your optimism and keep your spirits up. The following suggestions should help.

Excuses, Excuses

Most people have a standard set of excuses they use to "permit" them-selves to give in to external eating cues when they aren't physically hungry. Do any of these sound familiar?

- "I stuck to my diet so well yesterday, I felt I *deserved* that piece of cheese-cake today."
- "I was feeling so low that I really *needed* the guacamole and corn chips to cheer me up."
- "I *had* to sample the spaghetti sauce to make sure the spices were all right. After all, the rest of the family shouldn't suffer just because I'm dieting."
- "So what if I had a few brandy Alexanders after dinner? It was a celebration. Besides, I can always work them off tomorrow by running five miles and eating only carrot sticks all day."
- "It was Christmas."
- "It was Thanksgiving."
- "It was Washington's Birthday."

Behavioral therapists have found that recognizing your excuses can help you elminate them. Keeping your diary will help you spot the excuses you most commonly use. Once you've found them, organize them into a list. Then keep it with you, or tape it to your refrigerator door.

After a while, you'll find that the excuses no longer seem very rational or compelling. In fact, they'll probably begin to strike you as funny. When you can laugh at them, you've licked them.

Substituting Activity for Food

As I indicated earlier in the chapter, it's easier to eliminate eating as an inappropriate response to external cues if you substitute something else in its place. Otherwise, you tend to sit and fidget and fret about the food you're denying yourself.

The best substitutions are those that involve some kind of activity — something you can *do* to get your mind off food. Again, a list may be in order. Work out a roster of activities that you can turn to when the urge to overeat strikes. For instance: call a friend, take a hot bath, take a cold shower, chew some sugarless gum, take a brisk walk — anything to interrupt the act of reaching for food long enough to give yourself time to get over the impulse to eat.

Every time you're able to make a substitution, you'll have won a victory. This should make you justifiably proud and should bolster your determination to continue. And in time, you'll find that external cues will tend to prompt the activity you've substituted rather than the urge to eat.

An Expensive Proposition

Make fattening foods "expensive." Zero in on the high-calorie goodies you find especially irresistible, then agree to pay a friend or family member a small "fine" every time you eat one of these foods.

Don't make the fine exorbitant. The idea here isn't to punish yourself for being "weak," but to make you stop and think about whether you really need to eat — or pay for — that piece of chocolate cake.

This system can become an amusing game and at the same time make you more aware of your eating behavior.

Family and Peer Pressures

Family members and friends — well-intentioned or otherwise — can make a dieter's lot harder to bear. They may embarrass and undermine you by teasing you about dieting. Or they may insist, "You don't need to diet. You're not that fat." They often follow up such remarks by urging you to eat something you know you shouldn't have.

Many psychologists believe that teasers and phony sympathizers are motivated by jealousy. They may resent that someone else is able to make an effort to change for the better.

You needn't handle the hecklers and misguided reassurers by calling them liars or insisting that you *are* too fat. The best way to get them off your back is with calm self-possession. Tell them that while you appreciate their concern, your doctor wants you to lose weight and you agree with him. You might add, politely if possible, that you'd appreciate their helping you reach your goal by not making things harder.

Calorie Counting

Pocket-sized books listing the calorie content of common foods are easy to find. You can pick one up in any bookstore and in most supermarkets. It's a good idea to have one and to keep it close at hand, Make sure it is comprehensive and gives specific portion sizes ("4 oz., cooked," not "1 average serving").

The calorie counter will help you keep your diary accurately, but that's not its most important purpose. Its main benefit is that it will contribute to your sense of control over your weight problem. When you know how many calories you consume every day, you feel that you're controlling your food—not the other way around. This will increase your self-confidence. It should also make it easier for you to get back on the wagon if you slip off. When you feel that you're running the show, a lapse now and then won't be so devastating.

In counting calories, you're not only becoming more knowledgeable about the food you eat. You're also fighting two of the dieter's most insidious enemies—the sense of helplessness and the sense of guilt.

Relaxation

For some people, emotional stress is the most important of the external cues to eat. These are the people who turn to food for comfort when they're lonely, bored, frustrated, anxious, depressed, or distressed in some other way.

If you're in this category, you'll find that the best way to eliminate the stress-related eating is to attack the stress itself. In other words, learn to relax.

There are many relaxation techniques. Meditation works for some people. Yoga works for others. It won't hurt to shop around for a technique that seems right for you, and if you find one, all to the good.

But the relaxation technique that I recommend, and the one with solid scientific backing, is exercise. A good workout lifts your mood while it relieves your muscles of tension. Some psychiatrists have had great success in treating certain mood disorders, including depression, with exercise alone.

And of course, you'll burn a lot more calories exercising than you will meditating.

Joining Up

There's no need to fight your battle alone. Millions of other Americans are overweight and, like you, many are trying to do something about it.

TOPS (Take Off Pounds Sensibly), Weight Watchers, and Overeaters Anonymous are all reputable national organizations geared to giving you help and support in your weight-loss efforts. Consider joining one of them. Or join a diet or exercise class at your YMCA, YWCA, or local community center. Or call up your local hospital or university medical center and ask if they have a weight-loss clinic. Any one of these services may be of immense help to you. You'll get encouragement and support, and perhaps find new social possibilities, with people who have something in common with you.

THE NEW YOU

"The only way to lose weight is to make really big changes in your lifestyle," Dr. Stunkard once told *Time* magazine in an interview.

At first, this may seem to be an intimidatingly tall order. But as you undergo the process of retraining yourself, you'll probably be surprised and delighted to find that the new habits begin to seem natural very quickly. You're also likely to discover that you enjoy food more, while at the same time it becomes less of an obsession. Dieting becomes more of an adventure and less of an agony and a chore because you're concentrating on habits, not food.

As the habits change, a new lifestyle emerges to rescue you from the yo-yo syndrome and set you on the path of a sane, healthy, and permanent slenderness.

15.

EXERCISE AND WEIGHT LOSS

Fat people hate to move.

This may not be a universal rule, but it's an awfully prevalent one. Overweight people tend to be happiest when they're expending as little energy as possible. They'd rather lie down than sit, and they'd rather sit than stand. They'd rather read a book than walk around the block, and they'd rather read a hardback book than a paperback. Hardbacks are easier to hold open.

This is not to say that fat people are lazy. Their minds may be agile and active as can be. They may be capable of enormous mental effort. But study after study indicates that the obese seem to crave the comfort of inactivity, just as they crave the sensual enjoyment of food.

If you're fat, a suggestion that you exercise is probably about as welcome as a sentence from the Inquisition. Given the choice, you may very well prefer to keep the pounds and skip the agony. But before you make a final decision, give yourself a chance to be pleasantly surprised. Unlikely as it may sound to you, exercise could turn out to be one of the happiest pursuits of your life.

EXERCISE AND MOOD ELEVATION

I mentioned in the last chapter that some psychiatrists have been successful in treating mood disorders, particularly depression, by using exercise as therapy. Without drugs and without intensive psychotherapy, some dispirited patients achieve a much improved outlook on life after taking up regular exercise.

Unquestionably, exercise makes you feel good. After ten minutes of sustained muscular movement, most people begin to experience an elevation in mood. The high persists as long as the exercise continues and can last from six to eighteen hours afterward.

Moderate exercise — the kind you need for weight loss and the kind I'll describe in this chapter — is sufficient to make you feel exhilarated and cheerful. But should you find that you end up wanting more strenuous activity, so much the better. Dr. Robert S. Brown of the University of Virginia did a study showing that the more intense the exercise, the greater the high it produces. He found that runners enjoy the greatest mood elevation. Slow walkers, and mediocre tennis players whose movement is neither continuous nor intense, get no lift at all.

Scientists aren't sure why exercise improves your mood. The best guess has to do with the hormone noradrenaline, which you learned about in Chapter 6. Noradrenaline is a stimulant. People of an optimistic turn of mind tend to have high blood levels of it, while depressed people have low levels. Exercise can raise your blood level of noradrenaline to five times the normal level, and the elevation slacks off only gradually.

Whatever the reason, it should come as no surprise that exercise is good for your state of mind. Behaving in harmony with nature is the happiest and healthiest way to live, and exercise is natural. Being sedentary is not. From the days of the caveman, who had to catch his dinner before he could eat it, nature has meant us to use our bodies. A high level of physical activity is our natural legacy and our normal state.

WHY EXERCISE HELPS CONTROL WEIGHT

My bet is that once you've accustomed yourself to exercise, you'll like it very much. I hope so. For if you choose to be slender for a lifetime, then exercise you must. It's the only way.

Having read this far, you already know why exercise is essential:

- It's a natural appetite suppressant. As you learned in Chapter 7, exercise alters many of your own body chemicals in such a way that you feel less hungry. When you merely diet, you eat less because you make yourself eat less. When you exercise regularly, you eat less because you want less.
- It's the only way to make your body metabolically thin. It makes your hormones, your sodium-potassium pump, and your brown fat work in ways that encourage slenderness by maximizing calorie burnoff. You saw in Chapter 6 how exercise makes you burn more calories not just while you're working out, but twenty-four hours a day.

- It's the surest way to prevent the yo-yo syndrome. This is because of the three factors I just mentioned. Exercise is a permanent hunger-control device and a round-the-clock stimulus for calorie burnoff. Dieting is neither. Dieting is a state of self-imposed deprivation which, unless you're a masochist, is bound to be temporary. It does nothing to change your appetite permanently, nor does it alter your metabolism to help make you thin. Once you stop dieting, your appetite boomerangs on you so that you eat more, and your hormones encourage you to deposit much of that food as body fat.
- Finally, exercise helps preserve and protect your lean tissue while you're dieting. Losing weight without exercise means that 25 to 50 percent of the weight you lose will be lean tissue, no matter what kind of diet you're on. If you regain the weight, you'll regain it as fat, not muscle, and you'll be fatter than before.

MORE ABOUT MUSCLES

Before you begin designing an exercise program for yourself, an introductory word is in order about the muscles you'll be using.

Skeletal Muscles

When you think of muscles, you probably think of the bulging biceps of the body builder. And, indeed, the muscles that ripple beneath the skin of a well-developed body are one kind we'll be talking about in this chapter. These are *skeletal* muscles, or muscles attached to bones. Skeletal muscles are those involved in body movement.

Large skeletal muscles such as those in your legs and back are avid calorie consumers. They burn far more calories than fat tissue of equivalent weight. Suppose there are two people each weighing 200 pounds. One person is very muscular while the other is very fat. In the course of a normal day of only ordinary activity, the muscular person may burn as many as 800 calories more than the fat person.

You can see, then, that muscular people burn more calories in any kind of activity than fat people do. You also see why using skeletal muscles vigorously in exercise helps you burn a great many calories and lose weight.

Organ Muscles

Though skeletal muscles may be the kind most familiar to you, they're by no means the only kind — or even the most important kind — of muscles in your body.

Some of your internal organs, such as your intestines, are made up largely of lean or muscle tissue. Your heart itself is a muscle. This vital heart muscle must be strong if you're to exercise effectively. As you'll see, you'll be training and strengthening your heart with the same exercise that will help reduce your weight.

Muscle Makeup

Muscles are fibrous tissue composed of about 70 percent water. The remaining 30 percent is made up mostly of protein, with small amounts of fat and sugar. The protein that makes up muscles comes from amino acids in the protein food you eat.

You saw in Chapter 11 how muscle tissue is constantly losing and replacing its amino acids, and why you must provide for replacements with protein in your diet.

But eating protein provides only the raw material for lean tissue. *The main stimulus to assimilate the amino acids for use as new muscle tissue comes from exercise.* Without exercise, the building blocks for lean tissue can't be incorporated as readily.

This explains why dieting without exercise is so self-defeating. On a very low-calorie diet, your lean tissue loses amino acids rapidly. Since you're not exercising, there's little stimulus for the depleted tissue to replenish itself. Therefore, much of your lost weight will be lost lean tissue. If you return to your old eating habits and still don't exercise, the regained weight will be in the form of fat. You'll still be lacking a vital stimulus to put lost protein back into shrunken lean tissue.

How Much Muscle Do You Need?

The purpose of a weight-loss exercise program is not to give you big muscles and make you super-strong. It won't.

Muscles enlarge only when they're repeatedly and systematically forced to stretch at the same time they contract. Simultaneous stretching and contracting occur when the muscles are worked against *resistance,* or some opposing force. Resistance is the basis of strength-training techniques such as weight lifting. A weight lifter is making his muscles stretch and contract at the same time when he exerts his strength against the opposing force of a weight.

But the aim of weight-loss exercise is continuous, sustained movement — not sporadic, intense movement against some great opposing force. Weight-loss exercise does require some resistance. For instance, a runner meets with resistance from the ground when the foot strikes it, and a biker meets resistance from tension on bike pedals. But the resistance is a minor consideration, subordinate to the primary goal of smooth and constant muscular movement over a period of time. This continuous movement is the kind of exercise that makes you expend calories. It's also the kind that makes your muscles sleek, firm, and healthy, without making them huge or especially powerful.

Strengthening Your Heart

The one muscle you probably will strengthen considerably with weight-loss exercise is your heart muscle. It will become stronger as it adapts to handling a bigger workload.

The heart is a sort of muscular balloon. It expands to fill with blood, then contracts to squeeze the blood out through the arteries to the rest of your body. When you exercise, there is an increased return of blood to your heart from your exercising skeletal muscles. The greater volume of blood means increased resistance against which the heart must work as it contracts. The heart muscle is being stretched while it contracts, so it gets stronger. As a result, you're increasing your cardiovascular fitness while you're shaping up your body — another inducement to exercise.

ENERGY NEEDS AND CALORIE DEFICITS

Remember, in Chapter 13 I said you will lose *about* 2 pounds a week on a program that includes the Getting Thin Diet and moderate exercise. Some of you will lose a little more, some a little less. You will not all lose at the same rate, quite simply because you are not all the same person. Every individual is different, and no diet can guarantee exactly the same rate of loss for everyone.

Your exact loss per week will depend on how much energy you expend over and above the calories you take in; in other words, on your calorie deficit. Your deficit, in turn, will depend on five variables:
- Your size
- Your body's ratio of muscle to fat
- Your sex
- Your activity level
- Your age

The "Average" American

Remember our "average active American" — he of the 2,800 calories a day and she of the 2,100? Who are these fit people with their stable weights? And what do they have to do with you?

Obviously, the "average" American exists only in the statistician's mind. Each one of us is unique, so no one of us is likely to fit the "average" in all respects. Still, this mythical average creature can serve as a benchmark to help you gauge your own calorie requirements, so it deserves further exploration.

THE WOMAN

Our average woman weighs 130 pounds. She keeps house for her husband and three children, and she works as a typist. Here is how her day breaks down calorically:

In eight hours of sleep, she burns 440 calories. Even though she is virtually motionless, her living body is a hive of activity. Her heart is pumping blood. Her lungs are breathing. Electrical activity is going on in her brain. Her liver is busy clearing away body toxins and manufacturing new tissues. Her kidneys and colon are accumulating wastes. Her trillions of cells are pushing out sodium and taking in potassium. They may also be converting food to energy, or excreting wastes, or dividing to form new cells. Ms. Average may be doing nothing, but her body is using up a lot of energy just to maintain itself.

As she wakes and begins her day, her energy needs rise.

She engages in very light work for twelve hours. "Very light" means work that involves sitting or standing still. She types for about eight hours. For another four hours she may sew, or iron, or knit. In the total twelve hours, she burns about 900 calories.

She spends three hours doing light work. "Light" means work that involves some movement from one place to another. For instance, she may walk slowly to and from lunch. She may go shopping and carry groceries or packages. She may mop a floor. In these three hours, she expends about 450 calories.

Her remaining hour is spent in moderate activity. "Moderate" here — not to be confused with the moderate *exercise* you'll learn about later — means activity requiring more vigorous movement than light work. Our average woman may spend a few minutes walking faster than usual. She may spend some time scrubbing down walls, or enjoying some leisurely dancing with her husband. In her hour of moderate activity, she will burn 240 calories.

So we have:

Sleeping	8 hours	440 calories
Very light work	12 hours	900 calories
Light work	3 hours	450 calories
Moderate work	1 hour	240 calories
Totals	24 hours	2,030 calories

THE MAN

Our average man weighs 150 pounds and is an office worker. He is larger than our average woman, and is about 10 percent more muscular than she is.

In eight hours of sleep, he burns 540 calories.

For twelve hours, he does very light work. He sits at his desk, or he stands at home at his workbench drawing up plans for a new patio. In this twelve hours he burns 1,300 calories.

He does three hours of light work. He may weed the garden and sweep out the garage. This will cost him 600 calories.

His one hour of moderate activity may include mowing the lawn fairly rapidly, then lifting boxes as he cleans out the basement. In this hour, he expends 300 calories.

Our results:

Sleeping	8 hours	540 calories
Very light work	12 hours	1,300 calories
Light work	3 hours	600 calories
Moderate work	1 hour	
		300 calories
Totals	24 hours	2,740 calories

The Variables

If you fit neatly into the profile of Mr. or Ms. Average, you see where you stand in relation to the Getting Thin Diet, even without exercise.

Ms. Average needs 2,030 calories a day. If she eats 1,300 calories, she will have a daily deficit of 730 calories and a weekly deficit of 5,110 calories. She will lose something in the neighborhood of a pound and a half a week.

Mr. Average needs 2,740 calories a day. On 1,300 calories, he runs up a daily deficit of 1,440 calories and a weekly deficit of 10,080. He will lose almost three pounds a week.

If you aren't in line with the Averages, read about the following variables. Then use the chart on page 210 to give you a rough idea of your own calorie needs. Remember, every individual is different, so all figures are approximate. You don't need to pin down everything exactly; you just need to be in the right ballpark.

SIZE

One reason Mr. Average burns more calories than Ms. Average is that he is bigger. Body mass alone — even body mass as fat — is a factor in how many calories you need.

For a moment, view your extra fat with detachment. Think of your extra 20 pounds not as part of your body, but as a weight you carry around with you all day. For purposes of calorie expenditure, that's exactly what it is — extra weight that requires extra calories to maintain and carry.

Even though fat tissue burns little energy on its own, the extra burden it creates does change your energy requirements. For example, an over-fat 160-pound woman will burn almost 175 calories a day more than an overfat 150-pound woman, all other factors being equal.

Figuring how much energy each extra pound requires involves a complex set of variables of its own. For your purposes, it's enough to know that the larger you are, the more calories you need.

RATIO OF MUSCLE TO FAT

The more muscular you are, the more calories you burn, no matter what your activity level. Both muscle and fat create extra weight and mass that must be maintained and carried. But unlike fat tissue, muscle tissue is a big calorie burner in itself. Muscle cells are little furnaces that avidly metabolize food for energy. Fat-storage cells are exactly that — inert depots, for the most part. Because of this, muscles burn more calories than fat, even while you sleep.

Football players who lift weights to enlarge their muscles may take in as much as 5,000 calories a day without putting on any fat at all. But if they stay on the same diet after they quit playing football and lifting weights, they get fat.

No, their muscles are not turning to fat, as the conventional wisdom goes. What happens is that these ex-athletes are eating in their usual manner, but expending fewer calories on two fronts. They use less energy because they don't exercise. And they use less because their shrinking muscles are no longer burning the enormous amounts of calories they used to.

SEX

As you have gathered, size and muscle ratio add up to mean that men usually burn more calories than women. Men are usually bigger, and characteristically have larger muscles. You already know that the average fit American man has 10 percent less body fat, and proportionately more muscle, than the average fit American woman.

And as you'll learn in Chapter 17's section on strength training, men have an easier time enlarging their muscles. A man's muscles enlarge in proportion to how much he strengthens them. If he gets 20 percent stronger, his muscles get 20 percent bigger. But a woman must double her strength before her muscles enlarge visibly at all.

ACTIVITY LEVEL

I needn't belabor the importance of your activity level in burning calories, since that's what most of this book is about. If you exercise properly, you burn calories in the process, and you gear your body to burn more calories around the clock.

Let's look again at our 130-pound typist with her daily calorie expenditure of 2,030. Three sessions of moderate exercise each week will add at least 885 calories to her weekly calorie deficit. In one year, this would be enough to make her lose 12½ pounds, all else being equal, even if she doesn't diet. She will burn 250 calories in each workout, and her heightened metabolism after she starts exercising will contribute at least 45 calories more to the total.

With exercise and diet, Ms. Average's weekly deficit will be 5,995

How Much Energy Do You Need?

Individual calorie needs vary enormously from person to person. The following chart will give you a very rough idea of "average" calorie needs by sex, weight, and height, depending on degree of activity and exercise.

MEAN WEIGHTS AND HEIGHTS AND RECOMMENDED CALORIC INTAKE

CATEGORY	AGE (YEARS)	WEIGHT (LBS.)	HEIGHT (IN.)	ENERGY NEEDS (WITH RANGE IN CALORIES)
Males	11–14	99	62	2700 (2000–8700)
	15–18	145	69	2800 (2100–3900)
	19–22	154	70	2900 (2500–3300)
	23–50	154	70	2700 (2300–3100)
	51–75	154	70	2400 (2000–2800)
	76+	154	70	2050 (1650–2450)
Females	11–14	101	62	2200 (1500–3000)
	15–18	120	64	2100 (1200–3000)
	19–22	120	64	2100 (1700–2500)
	23–50	120	64	2000 (1600–2400)
	51–75	120	64	1800 (1400–2200)
	76+	120	64	1600 (1200–2000)
Pregnancy				+300
Lactation				+500

Adapted from Recommended Dietary Allowances, revised 1979, Food and Nutrition Board, National Academy of Sciences, National Research Council, Washington, DC.

calories — only 1,005 calories short of the deficit she needs to lose 2 pounds. In all probability, exercising three times a week will make her more energetic and more active even on days when she doesn't work out. The general increase in activity should be enough to take up the slack and allow her to lose 2 pounds a week.

As for our 150-pound man, he can expend 300 calories in a workout, and gain an additional 60-calorie dividend in increased metabolism. This means he will add 1,080 calories to his weekly deficit, for a total of 11,160. With diet and exercise, he will lose slightly more than 3 pounds a week.

AGE

Many people believe that their calorie needs decrease as they age, but this is not necessarily so. Your calorie needs decrease *only* if your level of activity decreases.

It is true that almost all of us will reach the point where we can no longer exercise as well as we once did. The natural aging process begins robbing our muscles of strength and elasticity when we're only about twenty years old. The encroachment is slow and gradual, but most of us can notice its effects by the time we reach forty.

Nevertheless, we do have a say in slowing the aging process somewhat. By exercising and eating properly, we can retain most of our fitness through our fifties and sixties, and even beyond. At the age of eighty, artist Norman Rockwell was still riding a bicycle five miles every day.

And the sort of exercise I'll prescribe for you is far less strenuous than five miles of biking daily. If you begin now, whatever your age, you should be able to achieve a degree of fitness that will keep your activity level, and your calorie needs, elevated into extreme old age.

THE KIND OF EXERCISE YOU NEED

Any movement is better than no movement at all. When you climb stairs at work instead of taking the elevator, or when you walk two blocks to the store instead of taking the car, you're burning extra calories. You're also training yourself to think in terms of greater activity. This is fine, as far as it goes.

But it doesn't go far enough. Physiologists have determined that the exercise you need for sustained weight loss and cardiovascular fitness must satisfy specific criteria. It must be:

- *Aerobic.* Any exercise is aerobic if it allows you to move continuously for an extended period of time without running out of breath. There's a list of aerobic exercises in the next chapter. All are good for weight loss.
- *Intense.* It's not enough to shuffle through exercise. To be truly effective, the exercise must be hard enough to raise your pulse to its minimal training rate. (See page 221.) This is the level at which you'll burn about 300 calories in half an hour. It's also the level at which you're recalibrating your metabolism and your appestat.
- *Regular.* You should work up gradually until you can exercise comfortably at your minimal training pulse rate level for thirty minutes, three

times a week. You don't really need to do more than this. But if you do less, you won't reap the full benefits of retraining your mind and body in ways that promote permanent slenderness.

• *Designed to use your large muscles.* Since it takes more energy to move your large muscles, your exercise must require their movement. Your leg muscles are the most important. Any effective exercise must give them a good workout. Your other large set of muscles is in your back. Exercises such as rowing and swimming, which work both the back and the legs, are excellent for weight loss.

The kind of activity just described is what I classify as *moderate* exercise. It is vigorous, exhilarating, and effective for weight loss. It is all you need to become a fit and slender person. After all, I'm not asking you to become an Olympic athlete. If you did aspire to athletic excellence, you would have to pursue more *strenuous* exercise. Strenuous exercise means putting more stress on your heart and working out for hours rather than minutes at a time.

If you end up liking exercise so much that you want to go on to strenuous workouts eventually, wonderful. But for now, let's begin at the beginning.

STARTING OUT

If you're overweight, you're almost certainly not a regular exerciser. If you were, you wouldn't have a weight problem in the first place.

If exercise hasn't been a part of your lifestyle, it's likely that you're out of shape in several ways, not just in regard to excess poundage. A major consideration is your heart, which may not be up to undertaking a moderate exercise program without some preliminary training. And your skeletal muscles may need some gradual conditioning before they're ready to handle the kind of physical activity that leads to maximum sustained weight loss.

Don't Be Impatient

There are overweight people who reach a critical level of self-disgust and then try to do too much, too soon. They should start with only a few minutes' exercise each day and build up gradually over several weeks to a full thirty-minute workout. Instead, they go out the first day and try to run five miles or swim forty laps.

These people often end up injured or disheartened or both. They may overtax out-of-shape muscles or an ill-prepared heart. As a result, they stop exercising, discouraged from ever trying again. Consider, for example, that 65 percent of the people who take up jogging programs drop out within six weeks, usually with injuries.

Don't make the same mistake. Go slowly. Be cautious. Be patient. It took years for your body to get out of shape, and it won't rebound overnight. You're not working for instant results that will fade as fast as they bloomed. You're trying to develop an exercise plan that you can live with all your life.

Don't feel you must accomplish everything at once. If you're on the Getting Thin Diet, you'll be losing weight by curtailing calories even before you begin to exercise in earnest. The purpose of the exercise is to accelerate the weight loss and, more important, to help you control your weight permanently. You'll get the maximum benefits in due time, *if* you don't foolishly risk injury by pushing yourself beyond the pace that's right for you.

You will know better than anyone else exactly what that pace is. Conditioning varies so enormously among individuals that it's impossible to dictate arbitrarily a precise point to start or a precise rate for proceeding.

But there is a rule of thumb: *Listen to your body when you exercise. Never push yourself to the point of being short of breath. Stop at the first hint of fatigue or discomfort, even if you've only been exercising for two or three minutes.* There's always tomorrow, and every day should find you able to do a little more than you did the day before.

Symptoms during Exercise that Could Mean that Your Heart Is Not Functioning Properly

- Pain in the chest, shoulders, arms, or abdomen
- Irregular heart beat
- A sudden very fast heart rate
- Shortness of breath when you aren't exercising very hard
- Unexplained dizziness
- Fainting
- Nausea
- Shortness of breath two minutes after easy exercise
- A pulse rate greater than 140 ten minutes after exercise

Cardiac Risk Factors that Indicate a Possible Need for a Stress Test

- Obesity
- Chest pain, particularly during exertion
- Irregular heartbeats
- High blood pressure
- High blood-fat levels
- A family history of heart attacks
- A resting pulse rate of more than 80 beats a minute (resting pulse taken upon first awakening in the morning)
- Concern that you may have cardiovascular problems of any kind
- Diabetes
- Kidney disease
- Smoking

Get a Checkup

Almost every weight-loss book tells you to see a doctor before starting whatever program it recommends. Sometimes the advice is sincere. Sometimes it's there to help protect the book's author in case someone who goes on the regimen gets hurt by it. In either case, the advice is all too often ignored.

Please don't ignore it when I tell you that you must get a physical examination before you start any exercise program. I can't overstress this advice, or the risk of ignoring it. *Exercise can't seriously damage a healthy body. But to an ailing one, it can be deadly.*

Where to Get a Stress Test

- From your doctor
- From another physician to whom your doctor refers you
- Most hospitals
- Many universities with physical education departments
- Many local health departments

Note: If your heart is already damaged, it is possible to develop a heart attack during a stress test. However, in a properly supervised test, this is extremely rare, occurring in 1 case out of about 20,000.

For an overweight person, or someone who hasn't exercised in years, even moderate exercise can be stressful enough to uncover weaknesses that haven't surfaced before. This is true regardless of age, though you should be especially cautious if you're over forty. A certain amount of tissue deterioration is part of the aging process, and it makes you more vulnerable to injury from physical stress. Besides, the older you are, the longer you've probably been out of shape.

If you're overweight, whatever your age, your checkup should include an *exercise electrocardiogram,* or *stress test.* This test gauges your heart's performance at various levels of physical stress.

You should have it because overweight is in itself a risk factor for heart attack and heart disease. So are other conditions that often accompany obesity, including high blood pressure, high blood-fat levels, and diabetes.

A stress test will indicate how much exercise your heart can take and whether exercise may make something go wrong. But even this test is by no means foolproof. It's only a screening tool. If anything in your checkup raises any questions, your doctor may want to do additional tests. Follow that advice. And if it turns out that your heart can't sustain moderate exercise, accept the verdict.

Usually, however, physicians find that a prudent and gradual exercise program is indicated to improve your cardiovascular fitness and general health.

THE FIRST SIX WEEKS

If your doctor gives the okay, your next step is to pick some form of exercise you find enjoyable — or, as the case may be, not too distasteful. If you were a good swimmer as a child, or a good dancer or a good skater, try picking up the activity where you left off. If you have never exercised, the following chapter contains some suggestions for a starting program.

Some overweight people are a little self-conscious about exercising in front of other people. If you want privacy, it's certainly possible for you to work out in your own home. You can ride a stationary bicycle, walk or jog on a mini-trampoline, or use a rowing machine — all without leaving your den or living room.

If you don't want to invest in expensive equipment, that's all right too. You can jog in place, or you can put on some music and work up your own aerobic dance routine.

One solitary and inexpensive form of exercise I *don't* recommend is calisthenics. Calisthenics are individual exercises usually lasting about one minute each and done in a series. The problem is that there's usually a pause between each exercise. Pauses violate the rule that your workout must be continuous. Of course, if you can do calisthenics without stopping, fine. In essence, you'll be doing an aerobic dance routine.

Pacing Yourself

If you're over forty and haven't exercised in more than a year, you should exercise for no more than ten minutes a day in the first six weeks of your program. Whatever your age, if you're a chronically sedentary person it may well take you the entire six weeks to work up to just ten minutes. It may take longer.

Start out the first day of your program by doing your exercise at a relaxed pace until your muscles feel heavy or begin to hurt, or until you feel tired. When fatigue or a feeling of heaviness or discomfort sets in, stop immediately.

The symptoms probably mean that your skeletal muscles are not yet strong enough to withstand the force you're putting on them. The problem will take care of itself gradually as the muscles adapt to greater stress. Your muscles will get stronger, and they'll have less to carry as you shed your extra pounds.

Muscle Soreness
From eighteen to twenty-four hours after each of your first few exercise sessions, you may feel sore. Muscles have a way of protesting against stress they're not used to.

Physiologists don't know exactly what causes muscle soreness. All we know for sure is that vigorous exercise damages muscles in some way, and that they heal stronger than before if they're given enough time to rest between workouts.

One theory has it that damage takes place in microscopic "bridges" inside the muscles. Muscles are made up of tiny fibers, and the fibers are organized into filaments. According to the theory, the filaments are loosely joined together by tiny bonds of some sort. These are the "bridges." Muscle filaments slide back and forth against each other during exercise.

Some physiologists believe the sliding of the filaments causes slight damage to the bridges, and this in turn causes soreness.

Whatever the cause, muscle soreness is more a nuisance than a danger. It isn't a symptom of real injury, and it shouldn't cause you any undue concern. The best cure for it is to keep on with your exercise program. Your muscles will get stronger and more flexible, and the soreness will disappear.

MUSCLE PAIN

Don't confuse either muscle fatigue or muscle soreness with muscle pain. Pain is always a cause for concern.

Pain is a subjective matter, but I define it here as a sharp, localized discomfort that occurs during exercise and may persist afterward. It's much more intense and specific than sensations either of tiredness or soreness, and you should have no trouble identifying it.

Pain indicates injury. It tells you that you've torn muscle fibers in the part of your body that hurts. This is the "pulled muscle" you hear athletes talk about.

The cure for an injured muscle is time and rest. *Sore muscles improve with exercise. Injured muscles get worse.* You must never stress an injured muscle before it has time to heal. If you do, you'll aggravate the damage. You may continue to exercise, but only in ways that don't involve the injured muscle. The time to begin using that muscle vigorously again is only after the pain has disappeared. Even then, go easy until you're sure the muscle isn't going to protest the renewed stress.

BREATHING

Breathing is a good guide to how intensely and how long you can exercise.

When you're exercising at the right pace you'll be breathing deeply, raising your shoulders and filling your lungs with each breath. This is called *sighing respiration*. With this kind of breathing, you'll still be able to talk as you exercise, and you'll feel comfortable. *If your breathing becomes labored so that you can't converse normally and you feel uncomfortable, stop at once.*

Some of you — particularly you smokers — may find as you start your program that the slightest exertion will make you short of breath. This means that your heart and lungs aren't up to handling the increased demand for oxygen that exercise imposes.

Take this as a warning to proceed very, very slowly. It's all right to breathe deeply. But it is definitely *not* all right to push yourself to the point where you're gasping for breath, at least at the beginning. To do so is to risk overtaxing an out-of-condition heart.

In the beginning, you may find that you can't exercise even for one minute without gasping for breath or feeling muscle fatigue. Don't be discouraged. You're not alone. Go as slowly as you need to, but don't give up. Once you can exercise comfortably for one minute, try for two — then three, then four, and so on. It may take time for you to work up to ten minutes, but getting there safely is much more important than getting there fast.

YOUR PULSE

A rule of physiology called the *Breckenridge Reflex* states that the more the heart is stretched, the faster it will beat. This means that we can take the pulse to measure how much the heart is stretching. This in turn shows how hard the heart is working. And in turn that shows how hard you're exercising.

You may want to use that tidbit to impress your friends at cocktail parties. Otherwise, you can forget it. The main thing you should know about taking your pulse during exercise is that you don't have to bother with it. Your body will tell you all you need to know about how hard you're working.

Sighing respiration is the key. The exercise will be increasing your body's need for oxygen, so you'll lift your shoulders and take deep breaths. No gasping or panting — just deep, comfortable breathing. When you're breathing this way, you're exercising effectively.

Here let me reemphasize: if you can't talk while you're exercising, you're pushing too hard. Panting indicates that you're near or at your maximum pulse, the fastest rate your heart can sustain without malfunctioning. You don't need to go this far for fitness or weight loss, and to do so can endanger an out-of-shape heart.

However, there's one pulse you should know about — your resting pulse. Your resting pulse is the rate at which your heart beats when you're completely at rest. The best time to take it is when you first wake up in the morning. This is the time when no stress or movement has had a chance to influence your heart's performance.

A resting pulse of 80 or above indicates that your heart is in woefully bad shape. Studies show that if you have a resting pulse this high, you're three to five times more likely to have a heart attack than someone with a resting pulse below 80. You must proceed very gradually, and only with your doctor's approval, to strengthen your heart. You may only be able to start out with a minute or two of exercise a day. No matter how short the session, be sure to stop at once when your breathing becomes labored.

The resting pulse can tell you when you've overdone your training the previous day. If it is 5 beats more than its usual level, you should cut back on your exercising that day, or even take the day off.

The resting pulse can also be used to tell you the absolute minimum of effort you must expend at exercise for it to have any training effect on your heart at all. If your heart rate doesn't increase by at least 20 beats a minute over your resting pulse while exercising, you will not strengthen your heart.

As your cardiovascular fitness improves, your resting pulse should drop. You can monitor it at least once a week to see if it's getting lower.

How Often?

How often you're able to exercise in the course of a week depends on how long it takes for your skeletal muscles to recover from each session. This depends in turn on what kind of shape you're in and how hard you're able to exercise each time you try.

Being overweight usually means that you're a real exercise novice. In this case, you won't have the strength and stamina to put any real stress on your muscles for the first six weeks or so. You'll be building up your cardiovascular fitness and the strength of your skeletal muscles in a very gradual way.

At any rate, don't exercise more than once a day. But do not exercise less than three times a week.

It's perfectly possible that you'll hate every minute of every session right at first. But I predict you'll be gratified at how fast you'll improve and how soon you'll be able to extend your workouts, expending more and more calories as you go.

If you can stick with a program for the first month and a half, you'll find the rewards are more than worth it. Your looks and health will be improving, and your spirits will be high.

TRAINING

Let's say that you've now reached the point where you can exercise comfortably for ten minutes a day. You've been dieting and burning extra calories, so you're already thinner. You've firmed up your muscles a bit, so you look slimmer still. Your muscles are stronger and they're carrying less weight, so the exercise is getting easier and more pleasant all the time. You're feeling cheerful and scrappy, and you're ready to take on new challenges.

Now is the time for you to start working toward the exercise pattern you'll live with for a lifetime, the thirty-minute aerobic workouts three times a week.

Duration vs. Intensity

If you're a novice exerciser, regardless of your age or weight, there's a general rule to help you set your workout goals: *Duration is more important than intensity. Your first aim is to extend the length of your workout, no matter how slowly or lightly you have to work to do it. Intensity will come later.*

Exercising at a relaxed pace for a longer period of time burns more calories than working feverishly for only a few minutes. Taking it slow and striving for duration before intensity is also the safest way to train. It gives your heart and muscles a chance to strengthen gradually.

So, as you work toward your goal of a half-hour workout, gradually increase the time you spend exercising, in increments of a few minutes each.

What Is a Workout?

Having thrown around the word *workout* a lot, perhaps it's time I tell you what one is.

For our purposes, a workout is the time you spend exercising with your pulse elevated to its minimal training rate.

The *minimal training pulse* rate represents 60 percent of your *maximum pulse* rate, which is the fastest the heart can beat and still pump blood effectively. The training pulse is the level exercise physiologists find is best for training your heart and for losing weight.

How to Calculate your Minimal Training Pulse Rate

AGE	MAXIMUM HEART RATE	MINIMAL TRAINING PULSE
10	210	130
20	200	120
30	190	115
40	180	110
50	170	102
60	160	96
70	150	90
Over 70		Raise pulse rate at least 20 beats a minute over resting pulse rate

Your minimal training pulse rate is 60 percent of your maximum heart rate.

Your maximum heart rate is the fastest that your heart can beat and still pump blood. It varies from person to person but a close approximation is obtained by use of the formula:

Maximum heart rate = 220 minus your age

The minimal training pulse is the recommended rate to strengthen your heart. It drops as you get older because your heart muscle fiber, like all your other muscle fibers, loses elasticity and can be trained with less force on it.

Anyone with a healthy heart can exercise beyond his or her minimal pulse rate, but it is not necessary to do this for fitness. Exercise physiologists consider 120 beats a minute a good training pulse for healthy persons of all ages.

Why Three Times a Week?

Every time you exercise, your muscles are injured slightly. It takes about forty-eight hours for them to heal. Exercising vigorously, before your muscles have healed completely, increases your changes of injuring them.

World-class athletes follow the forty-eight-hour recovery rule. For example, top runners will run faster on one day and more slowly on the next. They may run more than twenty miles on their easy days, but they will run them more slowly. Most top weight lifters lift only on alternate days. On their easy days, they usually ride a bicycle or run.

If great athletes require forty-eight-hour recoveries, so should you. Your first goal is gradually to work up to the point where you can exercise for thirty minutes every other day. That may be all that you want to do. If you want to do more, pick another sport for your recovery days. Your muscles will recover on the next day if you use them differently. For example, you could ride a stationary bicycle on Monday, Wednesday, and Friday, and swim on Tuesday, Thursday, and Saturday.

Why Thirty Minutes?

Benefits improve greatly when you go from ten- or twenty-minute workouts to a full thirty minutes. Stretching the half hour to a full hour will burn more calories, but the results are less dramatic than those of your previous step-ups in terms of fitness and weight loss.

Does this mean that the ideal exercise session lasts for thirty minutes from start to finish?

No. The entire session should last about forty-five minutes. The extra fifteen minutes consist of warming up, stretching, and cooling down — techniques I'll describe in the next section. The thirty-minute workout itself is the time you spend working hard enough to keep your pulse elevated to the proper training level.

THE EXERCISE ROUTINE

Every exercise session should consist of four parts:
- Warm-up
- Stretching
- Workout
- Cool-down

The warm-up must come first. Stretching can either follow the warm-up or follow the cool-down, but must never be done first.

Warming Up

Warming up means using your muscles at a relaxed pace in the same way you'll be using them in your actual workout. Warming up does *not* mean doing calisthenics or any other kind of exercise that fails to concentrate on the particular muscles you're about to stress. You warm up for running by running slowly, for swimming by swimming slowly. Here's why:

When a muscle is exercised, the blood vessels linking that muscle to the heart widen, increasing the muscle's blood supply. The blood carries oxygen to facilitate the efficient burning of glycogen, or muscle sugar, so you can exercise longer. It also warms the muscle, thereby making it more pliant and resistant to injury. When you exercise muscles at a relaxed pace, their temperature rises from about 98 degrees Fahrenheit to more than 100 degrees.

Light warm-up that exercises the same muscles you'll be using more vigorously later maximizes the warming and oxygenation of those specific muscles. In this way, it helps protect you and helps intensify and extend your workout.

Warming up also helps to protect your heart from developing irregular beats during exercise. When your heart doesn't get all the blood it needs, its electrical system may not function properly. Exercise gradually widens the blood vessels on the heart's surface so that more blood can get through.

You should warm up until you just start to break a sweat. Sweating is your body's main mechanism for keeping your temperature from rising further. So the presence of sweat indicates that you've reached the optimum temperature for serious exercise.

For most people, the warm-up will last from five to ten minutes.

Stretching

You must stretch to lengthen muscles that you shorten with exercise. When exercised muscles go through their process of slight injury and healing, the healing process causes them to shorten. Unless they're lengthened with stretching, the taut muscles are at a greater risk of tearing.

The muscles you use most are the ones most in need of stretching. A walker or runner, for example, will need to stretch the calf muscles, while a swimmer will need to stretch certain arm muscles.

Don't confuse stretching with warming up. Stretching does not raise muscle temperature. Stretching can follow either your warm-up or your cool-down, but it must *never* begin your exercise session. Stretching cold muscles is a good way to injure them.

We find hot baths relaxing because heat loosens taut muscles. The same thing applies to muscles warmed internally by increased flow of blood. Cold muscles are contracted and tight. Warm muscles are relaxed and flexible. Just as an overstrung violin string may break when a bow is applied, muscles that are cold and tight can tear under the stress of stretching.

A Stretching Routine for Back and Shoulders

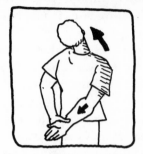

1. *Neck and shoulder stretch:* Put your right arm behind your back and grab that hand with your left hand. Try to keep the elbow straight and pull the arm over to the left as far as you can without hurting yourself, bending your head to the left at the same time. Hold to the count of 10 and then let go.

   Repeat 10 times and then do the other arm.

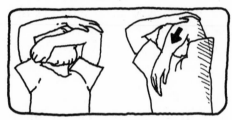

2. *Triceps stretch:* Stand up and raise your right arm over your head. Bend the elbow so your right hand rests on your left shoulder. Now grab the elbow with your left hand and *gently* pull the elbow over to the left. Hold for 10 seconds, then let go. Repeat 10 times.

   Repeat the exercise with the other arm.

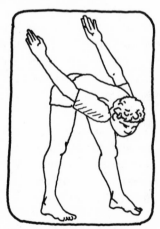

3. *Biceps stretch:* Stand with feet apart and hands at sides, with the palms facing backward, thumbs closest to your body. Bend forward as far as you can go, keeping your knees straight. Slowly raise your hands over you as far apart and as high as you can, keeping your palms facing backward.

   Hold for a count of 10, then return to your original position. Repeat 10 times.

A Stretching Routine for Legs

You need to do only four stretches to cover the four large muscle groups in your legs.

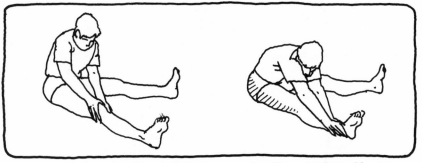

1. *To stretch the hamstrings in the back of your upper legs:* Sit on the floor with your knees straight and your feet widely separated. Put both hands on the same knee and slowly move your hands down your leg toward your ankle. Go no farther than you can hold for 10 seconds without hurting. Then let go, return to your original position, and repeat on other leg.

    Repeat 10 times on each leg.

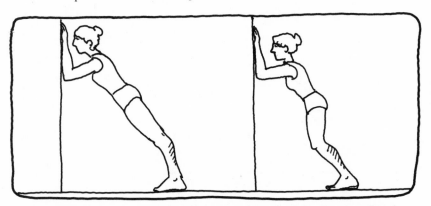

2. *To stretch the calves in the back of your lower legs:* Stand 4 feet from a wall and face it. Put your hands on the wall at shoulder height. By bending your elbows, you will bring your upper body closer to the wall. By keeping your heels on the floor, you will stretch your calves.

    Hold for 10 seconds and slowly release.

    This exercise should be done both with your knees straight and with them bent slightly. The two different knee positions will allow you to stretch different muscles. With your knees straight, you will stretch the gastrocnemius, your superficial calf muscle. With your knees bent, you will stretch the soleus muscle underneath the gastroc.

    Repeat this exercise 5 times in each position, as shown above.

A Stretching Routine for Legs (continued)

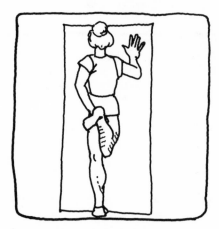

3. *To stretch the quadriceps muscles in the front of your thighs, and your shin muscles:* Stand up with your right knee bent. Grab the ankle of that leg from the back with your left hand. Slowly pull the ankle up and back and keep your knees together. Hold for the count of 10, then let go.

   Repeat 10 times, then repeat with other leg.

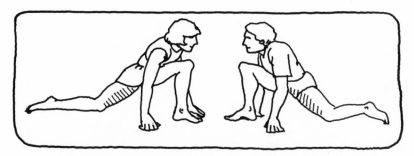

4. *To stretch the inner thigh muscles:* Stand up and slowly lower your body by placing one foot forward and the other backward. Continue to lower yourself until the knee of your forward leg is directly over your ankle, but stop at the point where it starts to hurt. The knee of your other leg should touch the floor. Then lower pelvis as far as you can without feeling pain. Hold to the count of 10 and repeat 10 times.

   Repeat with other leg.

Note: Shaded portions in the drawings indicate areas of stretch.

The preceding drawings have been adapted from *Stretching* © 1980 by Bob Anderson, Shelter Publications/Random House.

Always stretch a muscle slowly and smoothly. Do not jerk it, and do not stretch it farther than you can hold for a count of ten. Stretching too far and too fast instead of slowly and smoothly invites injury.

When you stretch a muscle too much or too rapidly, you activate receptors in its *tendon*, the "tail" that connects the muscle to the bone. The receptors send messages to nerves in your spinal cord, which relay back a message for the muscle to contract. A muscle that contracts involuntarily while you're stretching it is at risk of being torn.

Ten long, slow stretches for each muscle group that sees heavy duty in your workout are enough to keep the muscles pliable. Stretching should take you about five minutes.

Whether you stretch after warming up or after cooling down is a matter of personal preference. In either case, you're stretching warm muscles, but don't start a workout by stretching cold muscles.

Cooling Down

When you've finished your workout, you should never stop cold. Help your body get back to normal by cooling down. The process is similar to what you do in your warm-up. You continue with your workout exercise, but at a slower pace. You do this for about five minutes.

Cooling can help to dissipate heat from your muscles. It also helps normalize your circulation and minimize post-exercise soreness. As in warming up, you cool down from running by running slowly, and you cool down from swimming by swimming slowly.

THE "SECOND HEART"
When you exercise hard, your leg muscles act as a sort of second heart. When they relax, veins in your legs fill with blood. When the muscles contract, they push the blood back toward your upper body. If you stop exercising suddenly, your leg muscles stop their pumping action.

When this happens, gravity can cause the blood to pool in your legs so that there's not enough returning to your brain. You feel dizzy, and you may even pass out.

To make up for the sudden loss of your leg muscle pump, your heart has to work much harder to get the blood back to your head. This is no problem for a strong heart. But if your heart is weak, you can develop an irregular heartbeat.

By cooling down, you eliminate the leg pump gradually, and your heart is able to ease back into its normal routine.

LACTIC ACID

Cooling down can help prevent soreness by helping you clear a substance called *lactic acid* from your muscles.

Lactic acid is a by-product of glycogen that's burned incompletely because your muscles aren't getting enough oxygen to burn it entirely. When you use up a lot of oxygen with hard exercise, the lactic acid can build up in your muscles. It makes the muscles feel tired during exercise, and it irritates them and aggravates the soreness you feel the day after exercise. The longer the lactic acid is allowed to stay in the muscles, the sorer they're going to be.

Increasing the oxygen supply to your muscles by warming up helps delay lactic acid buildup, but it doesn't prevent it completely. Cooling down helps get rid of the lactic acid that does accumulate, by getting more oxygen to the muscles.

If you stop exercising suddenly, your heart rate drops immediately. Your blood flow slows, and your muscles get less oxygen, not more. But if you keep exercising at a relaxed pace, your muscles' demand for oxygen drops while the heart rate stays high. Oxygen is available to break down the lactic acid into harmless by-products, and your muscles escape unnecessary irritation.

And what do you do after you've cooled down?

Take a rest. You've earned it.

Recovery

Now that you're a regular exerciser, you may be so enthusiastic that you need a reminder about the recovery rule. It applies to all athletes, from novices to professionals.

Muscles get stronger through a process of injury and regeneration. But the regeneration takes time, and the time required is forty-eight hours. In other words, you should only do three hard workouts a week — or, at the most, a workout every other day. Doing more invites injury to muscles that haven't healed sufficiently to endure more stress.

If you want to be active on days off, fine. Just remember to go slow and vary your activities.

I can imagine what you're thinking right now. "Work out more than I absolutely have to? Me? No chance!"

Again, I predict that you'll surprise yourself. People who start exercising after being sedentary all their lives often report that once they get over the hump, they never want to take a day off. A good workout feels so great that on off days they miss it. "The hump," of course, is that first six weeks or so. But if you get through it and make exercise a part of your life, you'll wonder how you ever got along without it.

You'll look better. You'll be healthier. You'll be more energetic and optimistic. And you'll have the confidence and satisfaction of knowing that you won a major victory over your sedentary habits and your weight problem.

Recovery Pulse

Taking a recovery pulse can tell you when you've attained the fitness level you're aiming for.

But please heed this caution: *Never even think of testing your recovery pulse unless you know you're in excellent condition.* You must have your doctor's assurance that your heart is in good shape, based on a complete checkup that includes a stress test. And you must have reached the level where thirty minutes of exercise with your pulse at its proper training level is no problem for you whatever. A recovery pulse test involves all-out exercise, and it can be dangerous for an out-of-shape heart. It can theoretically cause a heart attack.

If you're sure you're up to it, you take your recovery pulse this way:

After warming up, exercise as hard as you can for five minutes. The idea is to push your pulse close to its maximum rate. Then stop and immediately put your fingers on the side of your neck, locating your pulse. Count the pulse for six seconds. Multiply the number you get by ten. This will give you your pulse rate for one minute. Rest for exactly sixty seconds, then repeat the procedure of counting for six seconds and multiplying the result by ten.

Your pulse should slow by at least thirty beats in the one-minute rest interval. If it doesn't, your fitness still is not up to par.

You can measure your improvement once you're well into your program by taking a recovery pulse once a month. The recovery pulse will slow as fitness improves.

Reversibility

Let's assume that I've convinced you. You're ready to gut it out and get into shape. You're even looking forward to it. But, you wonder, how long will you have to keep up the routine?

The answer to that one is, as long as you want to be slender and healthy.

Exercise isn't some magic trick that gives you a lifetime claim on the body beautiful. It's a habit that has to be permanently grafted onto your life.

If you get into shape and then stop exercising, a process the physiologists call *reversibility* sets in. Simply put, this means that you lose whatever benefits you've gained. Your stamina goes first, and it goes fast. Within a few short weeks, you'll find yourself panting if you try a workout that would have been easy only a month or so before. Your heart and lung capacity will deteriorate. Not long after that, your strength and speed will diminish. And — beware — the pounds will creep back.

Don't let this happen to you. The hard-won gains — and losses — are too valuable to lose.

16.

EXERCISES THAT WORK

"I play golf," you say. Or, "I play tennis. If exercise is so great for weight loss, why am I still fat?"

The answer is simple. You're not really exercising — not according to the definition of moderate exercise that you learned in the last chapter. Exercise that makes you lose weight involves continuous motion at your minimum pulse training rate lasting at least thirty minutes.

Yes, tennis can give you a fine workout. But only if you're up to giving John McEnroe or Chris Evert Lloyd a good game. Otherwise, you spend more time standing around waiting for the ball than you do moving. As for golf, the leisurely stop-and-go pace of the game renders it ineffective for meaningful weight loss. It may be fun, but it isn't exercise.

WEIGHT-LOSS EXERCISE

As you know, the exercises worthwhile for fitness and significant weight loss are the ones that get your pulse up to training level and keep it there for at least half an hour. These are the more familiar ones that meet the criterion:

Fast walking
Swimming
Riding a stationary bicycle
Riding a touring bicycle
Running (jogging)
Rowing
Ice skating
Roller skating
Aerobic dancing
Disco dancing
Walking or jogging on a mini-
    trampoline
Jumping rope
Cross-country skiing
Hitting a speed punching bag
Playing racquetball
Playing handball
Playing squash

Calories Burned in One Half Hour of Exercise

There is no way that you can compare the energy used in certain exercises unless you describe how intensely you are exercising.

For example, you can run at an 11-minute-per-mile pace and burn up 250 calories per hour, or you can run at a 5-minute-per-mile pace and burn 650 calories in the same time.

You could walk at a leisurely 3 miles per hour and burn 100 calories or at 5 miles per hour and burn 325 calories in a half hour.

The following table is for an average 150-pound person exercising without straining.

SPORT	CALORIES BURNED PER HALF HOUR
Lying, not moving	45
Walking	100
Swimming	300
Riding a stationary bike	150
Riding a touring bike	175
Running (jogging)	360
Rowing	175
Ice skating	225
Roller skating	225
Aerobic dancing	225
Disco dancing	250
Jogging on a trampoline	350
Jumping rope	400
Cross-country skiing	275
Hitting a punching bag	100
Playing racquetball	450
Playing handball	450
Playing squash	450

FOR OLDER PEOPLE, BEGINNERS, AND THE STILL-TOO-FAT

There's a lot of variety in the foregoing list, but not everybody has unlimited choices. You have to narrow your field a bit if you're over forty, if you're a novice exerciser, or if you're still more than 10 percent beyond your ideal body-fat level. (Remember, the ideal is 15 percent for men, 25 percent for women.)

Aging makes joints and bones more brittle, and it robs muscles of some of their strength and elasticity. In short, the older you get, the more vulnerable your body is to injury from physical stress. Of course, people age at different rates, and forty is not some hard and fast line of demarcation. You and your doctor may decide that, though you're past forty, you're up to taking on any aerobic exercise you choose. Nevertheless, forty is about the age at which most of us need to begin taking special care not to overstress ourselves.

What if you're a beginner — someone who has never exercised, or who hasn't exercised regularly in a year or more? You'll probably need some gradual conditioning before you're able to handle the kind of exercise that's best for weight loss and fitness. You're better off with an activity geared to gradual pacing, and one that doesn't require any new or demanding skills.

And what if you're still fatter than you should be? Your joints and muscles are already bearing excess weight, and they shouldn't be subjected to great additional stress. The extra weight is also making your heart work harder. You, like the older person, need an exercise that will give you a maximum workout with minimum risks.

If you're over forty, a novice exerciser, or a weight-watcher who has yet to get rid of enough body fat, these are the exercises I recommend:
- Fast walking
- Swimming
- Riding a stationary bicycle

These are the activities least jarring to joints and skeletal muscles. In fact, these three are often prescribed for people with arthritis. Many doctors also prescribe them for heart patients as soon as three weeks after heart attacks.

Fast Walking

The first good thing about walking is that everybody knows how to do it. You learn to walk early, and, barring a handicap or misadventure, you never lose the knack.

The second good thing is that walking is cheap. Your only investment is in a good pair of running shoes. (See the drawing on page 242.) Your clothing otherwise can be anything you please, and you can walk almost anywhere you want, admission free. As the mood strikes you, you can walk alone or walk with friends.

But perhaps the best thing about walking is that it's a minimum-risk exercise. It isn't likely to injure you. When you walk, one foot is always on the ground, so the other doesn't hit with a teeth-jarring thump. Your foot-strike in walking equals your body weight itself. This means that if you weigh 150 pounds, your foot bears 150 pounds when you take a step. Compare this with running, in which the force of the foot-strike equals more than three times your body weight. If you weigh 150 pounds, your foot hits the ground in running with a force of 450 pounds.

WALKING SPEED

For all its gentleness, walking can be a very effective exercise — provided that you do it fast enough. Slow walking isn't really effective for weight loss and fitness. It doesn't raise your pulse enough unless you're drastically out of shape, and it doesn't burn many calories. If you walk at the pace of 3 miles an hour, you burn only 66 calories. But if you increase the speed to 5 miles an hour, you'll walk farther and you'll more than double the number of calories burned per mile to 128.

But don't waste time trying to gauge your speed and mileage in walking. For you, walking fast means walking at whatever pace it takes to get to your training pulse beat and keep it there for thirty minutes. This pace is all you need to get you fit and trim, and sighing respiration will let you know when you've reached it.

Your conditioning determines how far and how fast you'll walk in your thirty-minute workout. If you're in poor condition, a short walk at only a moderate pace will raise your pulse to training level and possibly beyond. But as your fitness improves, you'll walk farther and faster at your proper training pulse. Alberto Salazar, the world record holder in the marathon, could no doubt walk fast for miles without getting his pulse beyond 120 beats a minute.

Start your walking program by walking at a slow and comfortable pace until you get tired or until your legs feel heavy or start to hurt. If you're not putting much stress on your muscles at this stage, it's all right to walk every day if you feel like it, gradually extending the length of time that you walk.

When you get up to ten minutes of comfortable walking, regardless of your pace, stop walking daily and start walking only on alternate days.

Work your way up to thirty minutes of continuous walking. Then start trying to walk faster.

In each workout start slowly, then gradually increase the pace until your legs begin to feel heavy or hurt or you feel tired. Then slow down. Pick up the pace again as you feel able to. Listening to your body's signals to determine when to push and when to slow down, you'll gradually achieve the ability to maintain a brisk pace throughout your thirty-minute workout. The same training level that once may have taken you only a block will now take you much farther, much faster, and you'll be burning plenty of calories.

BENEFITS OF INTENSITY IN WALKING

Walking has it all over running when it comes to the returns you get for increasing your pace. Running burns about 100 calories per mile, whether it's fast or slow. But with walking, you can more than double the calorie burnoff per mile by increasing the speed.

The reason for this has to do with form. In running, your upper body motion remains pretty much the same at any speed. But in walking, the form changes significantly as the pace increases. When you walk fast you twist your whole body from side to side. You raise your shoulders higher and swing your arms more. It's this exaggerated upper body motion that increases the number of calories you burn.

WALKING FORM

There's a proper form for walking as an exercise.

Land on your heels and push off on your toes. Take long strides. Keep your back straight and your toes pointed forward. Let your arms swing loosely and naturally at your sides. Don't hold them tight against your body; you'll only decrease your motion and tire your shoulders.

And hustle. Don't worry about mileage, but walk as fast and far as you comfortably can. Build up slowly, but reach the point where you can hold to the rule of walking with your pulse at training level for thirty minutes, three times a week.

Swimming

Whether you're fat or thin, young or old, swimming is a great exercise. It works the whole body, including the crucial leg and back muscles, to burn a great many calories.

Swimming is very easy on the joints and the heart. With the water helping to hold you up, your joints aren't even bearing all of your own weight. In addition, water buoyancy and your horizontal position when you swim make it easier for your heart to pump blood against gravity.

SWIMMING PACE

Intensity is important in swimming, as it is in any exercise. You'll benefit most in terms of calorie burnoff and metabolic fitness when you can swim fast and energetically.

But just as you don't gauge miles in walking, don't even think of counting laps in swimming. Again, the proper pace is determined by your pulse, not by your speed or distance.

The starting swimmer should follow the same rules as the starting walker. Swim slowly, extending the time of your session a little each day, or every other day, until you can swim continuously for ten minutes. Always stop as soon as you're tired or your muscles feel heavy or hurt.

When you can swim at even a slow pace for ten minutes without stopping, swim on alternate days only. Keep working to increase your time until you arrive at thirty minutes of continuous swimming. This is the point where you can begin working on your intensity, swimming a little faster for a larger portion of each workout.

As long as you aren't in very good shape, you won't swim many laps and you won't swim very fast in your half-hour session, even though the effort will elevate your pulse to training level. But as your fitness improves, you'll swim faster and cover more laps in the same amount of time and at the same training pulse.

Counting laps can be worse than useless; it can be harmful. If you set a goal to swim a certain number of laps, you may be less likely to heed your body's warning signs of pain or excessive fatigue or stress. If you ignore a muscle pain, you risk injuring that muscle. And if you gasp your way toward some arbitrary goal in laps, you may overtax a heart that isn't ready for the effort.

SWIMMING FORM

You can vary your strokes in swimming, or you can stick with the one that's most natural for you. Your intensity — not the stroke itself — will determine how many calories you burn in half an hour.

Whatever your stroke, the general rule for minimizing fatigue and extending your workout is to take full advantage of water buoyancy. Keep as much of your body in the water as you can.

Develop a kick that originates from your hips. This means keeping your legs fairly straight when you kick. If you bend your knees too much, your feet will break the surface of the water. This will slow you down and tire you more quickly.

Even your head should be in the water as much as possible. Keep it facedown in the water on alternate strokes. With every other stroke, turn it to the side just enough to free your nose and mouth for breathing.

WHERE TO SWIM

You don't have to have your own pool or belong to an expensive club or spa to swim regularly. Most communities have public pools where admission is either free or minimal in cost. Many YMCAs and YWCAs have indoor pools where you can swim all year for a very reasonable fee.

A lot of overweight people avoid swimming because they're reluctant to be seen in bathing suits. If this is true for you, try to get over it. Be proud that you're fighting to overcome your weight problem. And look around you. You'll find plenty of other people in the same shape. Meeting some of them, working together and comparing notes on techniques and progress, can make swimming a social pleasure.

Riding a Stationary Bicycle

Stationary cycling is a terrific low-risk exercise. The bike supports your weight while giving your legs a vigorous workout and burning lots of calories.

A stationary bike is much safer than a touring bike — that is, a bike that moves forward. You have to maintain a certain pace to keep the touring bike from tottering and falling over. But a stationary bike stays upright, allowing you to start out as slowly as you need to and work up gradually. And you don't have to contend with traffic.

A final advantage of stationary cycling is that the training it gives your legs is good preparation for skating and cross-country skiing, in case you ever choose to take up those sports.

The most important factors for stationary cycling are choosing the right bike, adjusting it properly and using it correctly.

Choosing the Right Bike

There are many stationary bicycles on the market, and some are better than others. Unfortunately, the bad ones far outnumber the good. Look for one that pedals smoothly when the resistance on the pedals is increased.

All bikes have some mechanism for increasing resistance. It allows you to adjust the tension on the bike to make it harder to pedal as your proficiency improves. But the cheaper models often have rubber or felt pads that rub against the flywheel to increase resistance. When you ride these bikes, the resistance varies throughout the full turn of the wheel. This makes you pedal with a jerky motion that tires you quickly and makes you more prone to injury.

To assure smooth pedaling, most good manufacturers use a very heavy balanced flywheel with a belt rubbing over the outside surface where the tire would normally attach. Other good models have vents on the wheel to catch the air in a way that allows equal resistance throughout the full turn. These are the bikes to buy.

Also be sure that your bike has toe clips that fit over the tops of your shoes. These enable you to pull up as well as push down as you pedal, giving your leg muscles the best possible workout.

A good stationary bike can cost anywhere from $175 to $500. This may seem steep, but you'll probably find the initial investment worth it. Your exercise apparatus will always be close at hand. You can exercise in privacy, if you wish, and you can divert yourself by watching television or listening to music as you bike. Or you can invite a friend to share the bike — and maybe its cost.

Adjusting the Bike

Once you have a good bike, make sure it's properly fitted to your body. It's important to set the seat high enough. If it's too low, your knees will bend too much, a situation that invites knee pain.

Begin adjusting your bike by putting one pedal at its lowest setting. Stand on it with your heel. Now set the seat so that when you sit on it your knee is just slightly bent. This should be the correct setting.

If the seat is too high, you'll know it when you begin to pedal. If your hips rock from side to side as you reach the lowest turns of the pedals, the seat should be lowered. Readjust it to the highest level that doesn't force you to rock.

Using Your Bike

When you first get your bike, don't tamper with the pedal tension at all. Leave it at its lowest setting. Start your program by pedaling against no resistance until your legs feel tired or start to hurt or until you feel fatigued. Do this every day, or every other day, gradually working up to ten minutes of continuous cycling against no resistance.

Still leaving the resistance alone, pedal on alternate days, working to extend your time to thirty minutes of continuous cycling. When you can do this, start working on intensity.

Begin your workout pedaling against no resistance for a few minutes. Then set the pedal tension slightly higher. Pedal until you feel tired, then lower the resistance again. As you recover, raise the tension once more. Try in each workout to extend the time you can pedal with the resistance raised.

Once you're able to get through the entire thirty minutes with the resistance slightly raised, set it a little higher.

As your fitness improves, you'll keep increasing the tension in increments. You'll also be gradually increasing the speed of your pedaling, in the same way a walker or a swimmer intensifies the pace of a workout. Before long, you'll find that you're getting a very intense workout and burning loads of calories. Just remember that in all stages of your progress, you're striving only to attain your proper training pulse for a thirty-minute workout. The fitter you become, the more intensity you'll require to elevate and maintain your heart rate at 120 beats a minute.

LATER ON

I recommend that most people over forty limit their exercise options to those I just described. But this caution doesn't necessarily hold for the exercise novice or the person who is gradually working off excess fat.

Suppose you're a newcomer who has gained the preliminary conditioning you need, or a weight-watcher who has brought your body-fat level to within 10 percent of the ideal. You've worked up gradually to a good level of fitness. You know you're in shape because you can get through your thirty-minute workout with no trouble. You're able to take your recovery pulse, as you learned to do in the last chapter, and the results are satisfactory.

At this point, you may find that you want to stick with fast walking, swimming, or stationary cycling. That's fine. Anyone of these will keep you healthy and help control your weight.

On the other hand, you may want to move on to something else. Here's a rundown of other possibilities:

Riding a Touring Bicycle

A touring bike isn't necessarily some ten-speed racing job. It's merely a bike that moves forward as opposed to one that stays in the same place. It's any sort of bike that you ride outdoors.

A touring bike gives you the same results as a stationary one, perhaps with more adventure and scenery — but with greater risk and inconvenience. If you fall off a touring bike while it's standing still, the short distance of the fall can cause your head to hit the curb or pavement with three times the force of gravity. This is very hard indeed. The fall can be harder and more dangerous still if the bike is moving.

If you ride a touring bike, you must wear a helmet to protect your head. You should also wear sturdy clothing that covers you up to protect against scrapes and cuts. If you do fall, don't try to jump free. Stay on the bike. You may lose a little skin, but you won't be as likely to break any bones or hurt your head.

Traffic is a constant hazard for bikers, and you should avoid it as much as possible. Seek out back roads or bike paths. Traffic also calls for slowdowns and stops that can prevent you from getting a thorough workout.

You can't ride a touring bike in your living room, of course, but you can make a social venture of it. Many towns and almost all big cities have biking clubs. Most of them have classifications that allow you to ride with cyclers of similar skill. These groups can be a great source of moral support. You can get a list of bicycle tours throughout the country by sending a stamped, self-addressed envelope to The League of American Wheelmen, P.O. Box 988, Baltimore, MD 21203.

Running

Despite its benefits and its popularity, running — and this includes jogging — can be dangerous for anyone who is not in excellent shape. It puts a jarring stress on your joints, and it's hard on your muscles. Runners make up a whopping 85 percent of the clientele of some sports-medicine doctors.

Another danger with running is that it takes you far afield. You may be several miles from home when you begin to feel tired, or a muscle starts to hurt. With no help close at hand, you have to get home on your own. This may be possible only at the risk of an injury serious enough to curtail workouts for several weeks.

On the plus side, almost everybody who gets into running and stays with it loses weight. The more miles you run, and the faster you run them, the skinnier you get, no matter how much you eat. The very form of running — bounding from one foot to the other — encourages continuity and intensity. As a result, running is one of the best possible exercises for burning calories and tuning up your metabolism. It's also rated at the top of the list of exercises that provide an emotional high.

Like walking, running is cheap, requiring only some good running shoes. And you can do it alone or with companions, in a variety of places.

RUNNING SHOES
Good running shoes are those designed to help protect you from injury.

There are two main factors that set you up for running injuries. The first is the force of your foot-strike. Your heel, landing first as you run, takes the shock of a force three times your body weight. The second factor is excessive *pronation,* or an exaggerated rolling inward of the foot as it hits the ground.

To help cushion the foot-strike, good running shoes have resilient, shock-absorbing material in the heels. Check to see that the shoes you buy have thick, well-cushioned heels.

Now for a word about pronation. When you run, you land on the outside of your foot and roll toward the inside. To an extent, this rolling is good. It helps distribute the force of your foot-strike evenly throughout your leg, thus cushioning shock and preventing injuries. But excessive rolling can cause your lower leg to twist too far inward. The resulting misalignment can cause injuries to your feet, ankles, knees, hips, and your leg muscles.

A good running shoe has features that help limit pronation: there should be a hard plastic covering, or *counter,* that fits around the heel. The heel should be flared so that it's wider at the bottom than at the

The Right Running Shoe

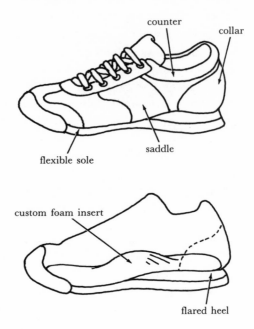

top. There should be an insert that is crushed down with wear to conform to your footprint. A *saddle* of sturdy material should run from the sole up to the area where the laces attach. All these features help stabilize and support the foot and hold it in place inside the shoe as you run.

Rowing

Rowing can be tough going, but it's one of the best exercises of all because it involves both the legs and the back. Remember, you burn the most calories when you use the largest muscles.

Rowing a boat is fine, but it's hard for most people to do on a regular basis. A rowing machine will give you the same results much more conveniently.

Be sure that your rowing machine has a seat that slides back and forth while your feet are held stationary. On this kind of machine, you have to use your legs to help move your body to and fro.

All rowing machines have adjustable tension for the bars that serve as "oars." You want enough resistance to make your muscles work, but not so much that smooth and continuous motion is impeded or that your workout is cut short because of fatigue. The tension can be increased gradually as your proficiency improves.

Rowing machines cost from $150 to $450. But, as with a stationary bike, you'll probably find that the benefits justify the cost. You'll have your machine available at your convenience for use in private and, if you like, in front of the TV.

Ice Skating

In order to burn calories and strengthen your heart, you need to build up your ability to the point where you can skate reasonably fast and hard. If you are already a skillful skater, remember that you won't burn a lot of calories doing figures in the center of the rink. Exercise means continuous motion, so go out and stroke around the rink.

Roller Skating

Roller skating can also help you burn a lot of calories, but the new polyurethane wheels are nothing like the ball-bearing wheels you remember. So be careful if you haven't skated since you were a kid. But work on building up your ability to the point where you can skate continuously for a minimum of ten minutes. Be sure you keep moving.

Whenever you skate, sensible precautions are in order. Roller skaters should wear bicycle helmets, along with pads for the hips, elbows, and knees. All are available at sporting-goods stores.

Aerobic Dancing

The popularity of aerobic dancing is soaring, and with good reason. It's an excellent exercise. It uses your whole body. It's rhythmic and entertaining, and it usually involves a lot of socializing with people whose goals are similar to yours.

Aerobic dance classes are sprouting up everywhere. Almost all health clubs and fitness spas offer them. If these alternatives are too hard on your pocketbook, check with your city or county recreation department for classes that are either inexpensive or free. If you're inventive and prefer to work out alone, it's also possible to make up your own routines at home. Books and records on aerobic dancing are available to help guide you.

Aerobic dancing may make you use muscles that haven't moved much for years, so it's possible that you'll be a little sore after the first few sessions. Don't overdo it. Observe the forty-eight-hour recovery rule. But do stay with it. It's a first-class exercise.

The only word of caution here applies to women who wear high heels a lot. High heels pitch your weight forward, causing an abnormal shortening of your calf muscles. Take care to work at stretching the calf muscles and strengthening the opposing shin muscles. Otherwise, you may wind up with shin splints — bad pains in the shin muscles caused by their being overpowered by the calf muscles.

Disco Dancing

Disco dancing is also excellent. If you really move, you can burn more than 450 calories an hour doing it. And if you enjoy it, you'll hardly notice the effort.

If you don't know how to disco, take classes. You'll learn enough to have a good time and burn a lot of calories, even if you never get good enough to compete with John Travolta.

A warning: discoing is great for losing weight, but only if you spend a lot more time on the dance floor than you do at the bar. Alcohol is packed with nonnutritious calories.

Jogging or Walking on a Mini-Trampoline

Rebounding on a mini-trampoline is another form of exercise enjoying a well-deserved surge of popularity. Mini-trampolines can give you most of the benefits of running without the risks.

Jogging on a mini-trampoline is much safer than jogging on a hard surface. Because the mat of the little rebound platform gives with each step, your foot hits with a force less than half your body weight. This amounts to one sixth the force of your foot-strike when you jog on the road. And since you use the mini-trampoline at home, it's always easy to quit or get help if you hurt a muscle or overtire yourself.

Walking fast on a mini-trampoline is also good. The rebound effect helps stimulate your circulation, so you reach your training pulse very quickly. The rebound also pushes you to keep up a brisk pace. And you never have to leave your living room.

Although I enthusiastically recommend jogging or walking on mini-trampolines, I'm not in favor of jumping on them. Jumping on the mat with both feet puts a tremendous force on your joints and has the potential to injure them.

A mini-trampoline will set you back about $85 to $200. But again, it allows you to exercise year-round, regardless of weather, with convenience and privacy.

Jumping Rope

Jumping rope is fine if you can do it, but most people lack the necessary stamina. You have to spin the rope at least 80 times per minute to keep it from getting snarled. This means you have to jump 80 times a minute, a task equal to running a mile in 7 minutes and 20 seconds.

At this rate, only very fine athletes can jump rope for thirty minutes without stopping. And jumping for less than thirty minutes is not ideal exercise.

Jumping rope is also very hard on the shins. Women who habitually wear high heels and do not stretch are more likely to develop shin splints.

Cross-Country Skiing

This is a wonderful exercise, requiring sustained movement against resistance over a long period of time. But it's not for everybody. You need the proper terrain and climate, as well as training, special skill, and a lot of stamina. It's just not feasible for most people to go cross-country skiing three times a week.

Downhill skiing is no substitute, no matter how much of a ski enthusiast you are. In downhill, the time you spend in motion on the slope is a tiny fraction of the time it takes you to get back to the top of the hill for another run. In other words, downhill skiing isn't continuous enough to satisfy the criterion for good weight-loss exercise.

Hitting a Speed Punching Bag

The big plus of this exercise is that it gets your pulse up to training level in a hurry. You do much of the work with your arms, and this makes your heart work harder. Your heart has to work two and a half times as hard to pump blood through the small vessels of your arms as it does to pump the same amount through the larger vessels in your legs.

Hitting the bag isn't the best possible leg workout, although you are standing and moving around to some extent. The compensation in terms of calorie burning comes from using big muscles in your back and shoulders vigorously and quickly. The rapid rhythm of the bag dictates your own rhythm, and you have to punch fast to keep up. A speed bag offers great continuity, once you get the hang of it, and it's very safe.

You'll pay from $50 to $100 for a lightweight air bag mounted on a metal base. You probably will also want to buy gloves. You can punch barehanded, but gloves help protect your hands against blisters and scrapes.

By the way, ladies, this exercise is not necessarily for men only. You may be surprised to hear that some women have entered the lists of professional boxing. Even though you may not want to follow their lead, working out with a punching bag is good exercise. And it helps train your eye-hand coordination to improve your performance in some other good weight-loss sports, such as handball and racquetball.

Racquetball, Handball, and Squash

As you'll hear again in the next chapter, the average tennis player lacks the skill to make the game a good weight-loss exercise. You get continuous, intense movement from tennis only if you're able to run down and return a high percentage of the balls that come your way. If you're not that skilled but you still want a racquet game, try racquetball.

Racquetball requires much less skill than tennis. All you have to do is hit the ball off any wall or off the ceiling of the racquet court. With no special training, you'll probably be able almost from the start to keep the ball in play enough to maintain your training pulse for thirty minutes. If you keep going an hour, you'll burn more than 900 calories.

Although perhaps less popular than racquetball, the related sports of handball and squash are equally good for losing weight.

Still sold on tennis? Or perhaps you think doing housework or enjoying an active sex life gives you all the exercise you need. The next chapter should change your mind.

17.

WORTHLESS WORKOUTS – AND WORSE

If you've been "exercising" with good intentions but no results, consider the possibility that you haven't really been exercising.

You may have taken up an activity that doesn't measure up to the standards for weight-loss exercise. If so, you deserve credit for good intentions and for burning a few extra calories. But you aren't reaping the full benefits of proper exercise, especially in terms of metabolic fitness and appetite control.

On the other hand, you may be relying on some gimmick or regimen that promises to trim you down without making you do any work yourself. You're worse off than the person who isn't exercising correctly. You're not only staying fat, you're being had.

Nothing you can do to your body from the outside — no heating or steaming or pummeling or pounding, no being jerked or jiggled by some machine — can make you lose fat.

What follows now are items that you should avoid if you're serious about reducing and controlling your weight. Some are ineffective for meaningful and lasting weight loss. Some are just ineffective, period.

SEX

"Reach for your mate instead of a plate!"

Sound familiar? It was the rallying cry of a weight-loss movement that was all the rage a few years back.

It seemed plausible enough. The idea was to turn to sex instead of food when you felt hungry. By replacing one pleasure (eating) with another (making love), you were supposed to stay happy and get thin at the same time. Along with curbing your appetite, all that sex was supposed to help you burn a lot of calories.

The first problem with this approach is that most people want food a lot more often than they want sex. Say you get hungry three or four times a day. If you're going to substitute sex for meals, you need a sexual partner who's always ready, willing, and nearby. Three or four times a day. Day in and day out. If you have that kind of laudable libido and bountiful luck, weight should be the least of your worries.

The second problem is the notion that sex burns a lot of calories. Forget it. Don Juan was fat. Cleopatra was fat. As a calorie-consuming weight-loss exercise, sex is a dud.

The Coital Calorie Countdown

Exactly how many calories can you work off by making love? With apologies to romantics, here is a step-by-step breakdown from kissing to orgasm.

KISSING

A kiss can use up about 12 calories. But that's only if you go at it with the gusto of Rhett assaulting Scarlett on the road to Tara. Otherwise, it's only about a six-calorie happening.

In general, kissing your loved one enthusiastically twice a day may allow you to lose one pound of fat a year, all else being equal in terms of food and exercise. If you figure in birthdays, anniversaries, and passionate reconciliations after fights, you might push that up to two pounds a year. That's if you forgo champagne dinners with your celebrations.

FOREPLAY

Things don't get much better as you proceed to more serious business. From a calorie standpoint, foreplay is hardly worth the bother.

If you keep at it for one hour you've proved that you're a great lover, but you've burned only 100 calories. It doesn't matter whether you're active or passive. A measly 100 is still the upper limit.

INTERCOURSE

In the real thing, enthusiasm does count. Just before orgasm and during thrusting, the aggressor burns some 250 calories per hour while the passive partner burns about 100. But how many people can prolong the actual act for a whole hour? Hardly any. According to the famous Kinsey Report, most men reach orgasm with only two minutes of thrusting. Women, if they're stimulated enough before thrusting begins, climax in about seven minutes.

Suppose you're a really exceptional lover who can make love aggressively for fifteen minutes. You'll burn 63 calories.

Even in intercourse, duration counts more than intensity. In other words, you burn more calories by extending your love-making than by performing it athletically. Not that it matters much either way, since the calories burned are pathetically few.

ORGASM

Ah, but orgasm. In orgasm you burn calories at the glorious rate of 400 per hour.

The catch, of course, is that orgasm doesn't last an hour, not even in the most lurid novels. It lasts about fifteen seconds. This means you have to divide 400 by 240, for a grand total of 1.6 calories per orgasm. Think of it as about one thirteenth of a cup of asparagus.

Don't bother with all the math. The long and short of it is this: if you're a magnificent lover going full-tilt for an hour, you're using up only about 250 calories. If you're a magnificent, aggressive lover who's madly in love and somewhat oversexed, it's just possible that you can lose 25 pounds in a year. That's provided that you have sex *con brio* at least once a day. And it applies only if you eat no more than usual and stay as active vertically as you are horizontally.

MASSAGE

Like sex, massage is a wonderful sensual experience. But massage is even less effective than sex for doing anything about your weight. Sex at least burns *some* extra calories. Lying down while someone rubs and kneads your body burns virtually none.

Massage does help warm your muscles because of a physiological phenomenon called the *red reflex*. When pressure is applied to any part of your body, blood vessels in the affected area widen to increase the flow of blood to the muscles and skin being pressed. The blood-enriched muscles feel good, but they're not in use so they're not expending any extra calories. Nor are they getting any stronger or firmer.

And don't get the idea that increasing blood flow with massage does anything good for your heart. The increased flow caused by the red reflex is highly localized, transient, and minimal. There is no increased blood flow back to the heart, which is not stressed at all.

Finally, don't think that a massage might be a pleasant substitute for warming up before a workout. The slight, localized increase in blood flow from the red reflex doesn't begin to compare with the general circulatory increase that comes from using your muscles in a warmup.

PASSIVE "EXERCISE"

Some reducing salons offer machines that are supposed to take the strain out of exercise by doing the work for you. There are, for instance, tables that jiggle you around, belts that vibrate you, bicycles that pedal for you, rollers that pummel your flab. With such gadgets, the machine has a better chance of losing weight than you do. After all, it's doing all the work.

You can't lose weight without burning calories, and you can't burn calories without expending effort. No machine can substitute for your own hard work. Don't kid yourself. They're useless.

SPOT "REDUCING"

As I told you way back in Chapter 1, there's no such thing as spot reducing. Losing weight requires you to burn more calories than you eat, and you burn the most calories by using the most muscles. When you do lose weight, you lose it from wherever it was stored in the first place — which may or may not be in the area you're trying to reduce.

Therefore, it makes no sense to limit your exercising to a specific set of muscles in hopes of reducing the size of a specific part of your body. By limiting the muscles you use, you're only limiting the number of calories you burn.

It's true that muscles that get a lot of exercise will become stronger and firmer, but this does not mean that spot exercising will make you look more sleek. If you aren't losing weight, the thickness of the fat layer covering the muscles remains the same. Firm or not, the muscles aren't close enough to the skin to give you a smooth, attractive look.

If you're exercising against resistance in your spot-reducing program, you may get results you didn't bargain for at all. You may strengthen the muscles enough to enlarge them. If the muscles get bigger and the fat layer remains the same, the very spot you're working so hard to reduce gets larger instead of smaller.

Spot reducing has little value because it doesn't aim at reducing your fat. Remember, tennis players exercise one arm all the time, but that arm matches the other almost exactly in terms of fat content.

CALISTHENICS

I explained the problem with calisthenics in Chapter 15. Separate exercises done in a series are worthwhile for meaningful weight loss only if they're done without pauses. This is not how most people do them.

In the usual calisthenic series, you might do a few pushups, then stop to shift position for the next exercise. Then you do a few sit-ups and stop, then a few knee bends, and so forth. With every pause you allow your pulse to drop, so you're not obeying the continuity rule for good weight-loss exercise.

Another drawback is that calisthenics tend to exercise only a few muscles at a time. They don't require the continual movement of your large muscles, so they're less than ideal for burning calories. And they usually don't train your heart. To strengthen your heart, you have to exercise continuously for at least ten minutes. Since most people don't do calisthenics continuously, they don't train their hearts. In short, calisthenics are neither efficient nor effective as far as most people's basic exercise needs go. They may be better than nothing at all — but not much.

TENNIS

As I've already pointed out, tennis requires so much skill that only the best players can keep a rally going long enough for a real workout. The average player spends 80 percent of the time waiting for the ball. Standing around on a tennis court is no more productive than standing around anywhere else.

In an hour on the court, the so-so tennis player burns about 200 calories — a trifling number compared to the 650 calories you can work off in an hour of racquetball.

Tennis is certainly better for you than sitting around the house watching television, but that's about the best you can say for it.

GOLF

Golf is too sporadic and too slow. The only hard work it demands is taking a good swat at the ball, and you do this only from time to time. Walking around a golf course, no matter how fast, does little good because you stop so often. And in this age of the golf cart, who walks anyway?

CLIMBING STAIRS

Yes, climbing a flight of stairs burns more calories than taking the elevator. If you're presented with a choice, I certainly encourage you to take the stairs. Climbing them often enough will firm up your muscles a bit and reinforce your resolution to be more active.

But no, climbing stairs does not qualify as good weight-loss exercise — because, if for some strange reason they wanted to, few people could climb stairs for thirty minutes at a time. If your climb is any shorter, you're violating the rule that your pulse must stay elevated to training level for at least a half hour.

HOUSEWORK

I will not argue with the homemaker's contention that housework is hard work. But it's not intensive and uninterrupted hard work. Mopping floors and chasing kids won't satisfy the criteria for weight-loss exercise, not even if you have ten children and run a house the size of Buckingham Palace.

Besides, I've never met anyone who thinks housework offers much in the way of excitement. Housework is work. Exercise should be fun. You'll do a lot better staying with your exercise program if you take up an activity that is enjoyable and provides a break in your usual routine.

STRENGTH TRAINING

Weight lifting and other strength-training exercises are good for getting stronger, but not necessarily slimmer. Weight lifting is an intermittent activity, not a continuous one. Hardly anyone is strong enough to lift weights without stopping for thirty minutes at a time. The same is true of working against heavy resistance on strength-training machines such as Nautilus equipment.

Lifting a weight raises your pulse considerably, but the elevation is not sustained. Studies show that while world-class weight lifters can raise their pulse rates to more than 120 beats a minute with a single bench press, the rate drops to below 90 less than two minutes after they put the weight down. Since the exercise is not continuous, it burns comparatively few calories.

Of course, strength training can firm up and enlarge your muscles if you keep at it. Men's muscles enlarge in direct proportion to the amount of strength they gain. In other words, if a man becomes stronger, his muscles get bigger. So if he lifts weights or uses resistance equipment in conjunction with aerobic exercises that help him lose weight, he will have a body with attractive muscle definition.

Women can also tone and firm their muscles with strength training, but only a dedicated body builder is likely to enlarge her muscles appreciably. Mostly because of hormonal differences, women's muscles don't respond to strength training in the same way men's do. A woman has to double her strength before her muscles will visibly enlarge.

Though strength training is not a good calorie burner, it's not without value in a weight-loss program. Since muscle tissue burns far more calories than fat tissue, becoming more muscular will help you burn more calories in any activity, including aerobic exercise.

A word of caution: don't attempt any kind of strength training unless your heart is in excellent shape. When muscles contract hard against an opposing force, they increase the resistance to blood flow inside your blood vessels. As a result, your blood pressure undergoes a sharp and sudden rise. The strain can be dangerous for an ill-conditioned heart.

SAUNAS

Sitting in a sauna will raise your pulse, but for the wrong reasons. When your body temperature rises, your heart has to pump extra blood to your skin to help cool you. This causes your heart rate to go up. Your heart is working slightly harder than usual, but your muscles aren't working at all. The net result is that you're not burning enough extra calories to lose any fat. You are sweating off water weight, but it will return as soon as you drink fluid or eat a meal.

Like massage, sitting in a sauna is no substitute for warming up before a workout. A sauna does warm the muscles, but it does not increase the blood flow to them. A good workout requires the increased flow of oxygen-bearing blood that a warm-up provides.

RUBBER SWEAT SUITS

Working out in a rubber sweat suit is self-defeating.

More than 70 percent of the energy your body expends is lost as heat; only 30 percent is used to fuel your muscles. Sweating is the main cooling device for coping with heat buildup during exercise. As the sweat evaporates from your skin, it cools you.

Rubber sweat suits interfere with this vital temperature-control mechanism by preventing sweat from evaporating. You'll sweat more, as your body struggles against stacked odds to keep you cool. But the struggle will make you so tired that you can't get through a full workout. Since you exercise less, you burn fewer calories and retain more fat. The water loss you achieve reverses itself quickly as you drink to relieve your dehydration.

HEAT BELTS

This is a variation on the rubber sweat-suit theme. The belts are billed as devices that "melt away inches" from your waist. Some of the belts have chemical heat packs to increase the temperature around your middle to make you sweat more. Others are just elaborate elasticized waist cinchers that fit close and keep sweat from evaporating.

In either case, any loss of inches you get from wearing a heat belt is purely temporary. The dehydrated cells around your waist blow right back up as soon as they get the water they need.

Nothing melts fat except the surely lethal temperature of 360 degrees Fahrenheit.

BODY WRAPS

Same song, last verse. Some spas specialize in mummifying you in plastic wrap for a time, with assurances that this will melt off inches.

The wrap will make you sweat more, and you'll probably lose some water weight. You may even look slimmer for an entire night on the town, as long as you neither eat nor drink anything. Unless you're suicidal, however, you must eventually ingest some fluid or food. When you do, the lost inches come right back.

Body wraps are among the seemingly endless ways to a "trimmer you." Beware of easy ways. They almost never work. The only sweating that's going to help you lose fat is the sweating you do in a good workout.

BE WARY

As you can see, nonsense abounds about exercise and weight-loss gimmicks, just as nonsense abounds about diet. The weight-conscious American public provides a huge and tempting market for quick-buck predators who don't mind abusing their right to freedom of speech by bending the truth a bit.

There are also some exercise counselors who counsel the wrong kind of exercise. You're apt to find them here and there in the burgeoning but largely unregulated health spa business. Though perhaps less sinister than the gimmick makers, the counselors who strap you to vibrating tables or put you through worthless calisthenics aren't doing you any good. At best, you're being sidetracked from exercising the right way.

If you want to join a spa, you're now armed with the information you need to find a good one — one run by people who're genuinely knowledgeable about exercise physiology. Shop around and ask questions. If anyone offers to wrap you in plastic or put you on a self-pedaling bike, head for the nearest exit.

As for the gimmicks, they're good for a laugh as long as *you* don't waste your time and money on them. Treat them as the bad jokes they are, and let the laugh be on somebody else.

When you hear that some gizmo melts away fat, turn your back and zip up your pockets. You're among the lucky folks who know that when it comes to getting rid of fat, there simply are no substitutes for more active muscles and a less active mouth.

18.

EXTRAORDINARY MEASURES

There are millions of Americans who are mildly overweight, but otherwise healthy in mind and body. If you're among them, count yourself lucky.

You have a problem, but it's not unmanageable or hopeless. Just by reading this book you've come a long way toward solving it. You know enough by now to build a workable lifetime approach to weight control based on regular exercise, sensible diet, and a program to modify bad eating habits.

You're lucky because for you, these three methods should work. Apply them with determination and tenacity, and you'll almost certainly get thin and stay that way.

Not everybody is so lucky. There are, of course, people who will always reject conventional methods in favor of fads and gimmicks that seem to offer easier solutions. And there are the pitiable anorexics and bulimarexics, who use bizarre and dangerous weight-loss stratagems in their obsessive compulsion to emaciate themselves.

But perhaps the most unfortunate of all are the people who suffer from morbid obesity. For them, there may be no choice but to seek out extraordinary measures — perilous and extreme remedies that can be justified only by life-or-death necessity.

MORBID OBESITY

The word "morbid" in morbid obesity comes from the Latin *morbidus*, meaning "disease." And indeed, the condition is a life-threatening illness.

You are morbidly obese when your excess fat is sufficient to threaten your physical or mental health, or both, in a severe and imminent way.

A doctor would diagnose morbid obesity in a man whose body fat constitutes 50 percent of his total weight, or in a woman with 75 percent body fat. The term also applies if you are 100 pounds or more overweight, or if your weight is twice that proposed as ideal by insurance company actuarial tables.

If you are morbidly obese, you are so fat that you have no chance of living a normal life span. Your heart can fail because it lacks the strength to pump blood throughout your massive body. You can contract diabetes because your overfull fat cells can no longer respond to insulin, and your blood sugar skyrockets. Your immune system can fail, making you more susceptible to certain kinds of cancer. If you're a morbidly obese woman, your chances of developing cancer of the breast or uterus are far greater than normal.

The death rate for victims of morbid obesity between the ages of twenty-five and thirty-five is twelve times that of normal people in the same age group. It is sixfold between the ages of thirty-five and forty-five, and threefold between the ages of forty-five and fifty-five. The decreasing ratio does not mean that morbid obesity becomes safer as you age. On the contrary, the longer you have the condition, the greater the likelihood of death. The ratio decrease merely reflects the fact that the death rate for normal people increases as they age.

Causes of Morbid Obesity

People who suffer from obesity caused by a known glandular abnormality make up a small percentage of the morbidly obese. You'll remember that true glandular obesity accounts for less than 1 percent of all obesity. There are any number of complex hormonal irregularities that can cause glandular morbid obesity, but such cases remain the rare exceptions rather than the rule.

Glandular causes aside, scientists are not yet entirely sure why some people cross the line from moderate overweight to life-threatening obesity. It appears, however, that the morbidly obese have serious defects in the mechanisms that control appetite, or those that govern satiety, or both. In a very literal sense, their eating is out of control.

We also know that morbidly obese people have more than three times as many fat cells as other people. The average person has about 25 billion fat cells. The morbidly obese person has at least 75 billion fat cells, and in some cases even more.

It is possible that some morbidly obese people are born with an unduly large number of fat cells. As you know, some experts theorize that heredity may predetermine fat-cell number. You'll also recall that a fetus can become too fat while still in the womb from overfeeding on the high blood sugar of its diabetic mother. But in the main, the great proliferation of fat cells that characterizes morbid obesity is caused by uncontrolled eating.

Why Conventional Treatment Fails

Referring to the discussion of fat cells in Chapter 8 will help you understand the dilemma of morbid obesity. Trapped by fat cells and a badly flawed appestat, the victim is caught in a vicious cycle that makes a mockery of dieting.

You'll remember that fat cells can be emptied, but not eliminated. And empty fat cells strive to be refilled. They secrete the enzyme LPL that helps drive fat out of the bloodstream and into the fat cells.

Because of extreme hunger, the morbidly obese person cannot diet effectively for very long at a time. A short period of dieting only looses a flood of LPL from depleted fat cells. As the victim returns to overeating, the LPL helps see to it that as much food as possible ends up as stored fat. The fat cells quickly refill. In addition, lean tissue lost during the diet is replaced by fat. The net result is yet another escalation of fat cells.

Exercise is seldom the answer either. In fact, exercise is out of the question for almost all the morbidly obese, since even the slightest exertion might endanger their overburdened circulatory systems.

Since diet and exercise are all but impossible, behavior modification has no meaning for treating the morbidly obese. Sad to report, doctors have had very little success in treating such people with methods used to treat moderately obese patients.

The morbidly obese person faces a terrible dilemma: he or she has a killing disease, and it will not respond to conventional treatment in most cases. The choices are clear-cut and limited: radical treatment or death.

Surgery

Let me emphasize at the outset that surgery is never acceptable except as a desperate last resort for the treatment of life-threatening obesity. The risks are too great.

Certainly, no one should even consider an operation unless all conventional methods have failed repeatedly. In any case, a person foolish enough to seek out a surgical solution to a fat problem as long as there are any other options would be unlikely to secure one. No responsible surgeon will perform surgery unless all other possible treatments have been eliminated. All the surgical procedures dealing with morbid obesity are fraught with appalling potential side effects.

CHOOSING A SURGEON

Should you believe that you have no recourse but surgery, take great time and care to find the right surgeon. Most surgeons have no experience whatever in obesity operations. Besides, as you will see, some surgical methods are preferable to others. Some procedures that were common only a few years ago have been all but abandoned because their fatality rates were so high. And even the procedures still in use sometimes have such horrendous side effects that the surgery must be reversed.

One way to find a suitable surgeon is to ask your doctor to recommend one who is experienced in treating morbid obesity. If your doctor cannot make a referral, call a medical school or your local medical society.

But a better first step would be to contact a gastroenterologist. This is a medical doctor who specializes in the stomach and intestines but does not do surgery. Such a physician will usually know who in your community is competent to do the surgery and who is not — knowledge that comes from experience treating patients who have had varying degrees of success with surgery.

Once you find a surgeon, he will assess your condition and determine whether you are a candidate for surgery. If you are not entirely satisfied with the decision, by all means find another obesity surgeon and get a second opinion.

I should add here that a surgeon may not be the only doctor you should consult. It may be wise to see a psychiatrist as well. It takes a great deal of emotional stamina to face the pain that follows obesity surgery, and the other side effects that may ensue. In addition, the surgery occasionally involves such psychological aftereffects as confusion, depression, and drastic mood swings. A psychiatrist may be able to help you prepare for surgery, help deal with any complications in your recuperative period, and may also be able to help you decide if surgery is truly the choice you want to make.

TYPES OF SURGERY

There are three main categories of surgery used to treat morbid obesity:

- Surgery involving the intestines, aimed at limiting food absorption (*intestinal bypass*)
- Surgery dealing mainly with the stomach, aimed at limiting food intake (*gastric cutting* and *gastric stapling*)
- Surgery on the vagus nerve, which helps govern appetite (*vagotomy*)

All these procedures are relatively new. The intestinal bypass is the oldest, having first been performed in 1965. Stomach surgery followed a year later, and the first vagotomy was reported in 1978.

INTESTINAL BYPASS

There are at least ten different techniques for this procedure, but all are aimed at effecting weight loss by shortening the small intestine.

Your digestive tract is a remarkable piece of plumbing about thirty feet long, running from your mouth to your anus. It includes the mouth, the esophagus, the stomach, the small and large intestines, and the rectum.

A minute amount of food nutrients is absorbed into your bloodstream directly from your stomach. The large intestine, also called the lower bowel or colon, is the last stop for food awaiting elimination. The colon, about six feet long, absorbs water and some minerals from this waste material.

It is the small intestine that accounts for the absorption of some 99 percent of the nutrients and calories in the food you eat. Joining the stomach to the colon, the small intestine is only about 23 feet long. But it provides some 1,120 square feet of absorptive surface. This is because its inside walls are lined with tiny fingerlike projections called *villi*. In addition, each cell of the interior walls is lined with microscopic projections called *microvilli*. Blood vessels in the villi pick up nutrients from digested food and carry them away for use by your body.

The Procedure Scientists who pioneered the intestinal bypass reasoned this way: the small intestine absorbs almost all the calories derived from food. Therefore, one might drastically curtail the calories available to be stored as fat by shortening the small intestine.

The operation involves cutting the small intestine as close as two feet below the stomach and attaching the short piece directly to the colon. In this way, as much as 18 feet of the intestine may be bypassed. The bypassed section isn't removed. Its nerves and blood vessels remain intact, and it remains alive. It simply no longer carries, processes, or absorbs nutrients.

Early versions of this procedure allowed the bypassed section to lie unattached to any drainage site in the abdominal cavity. The result was that many patients died. They suffered liver or brain failure, presumably caused by poisons from putrefying bacteria in the bypassed section. The still-living section went on secreting enzymes and other fluids, even though it no longer received food. It appeared that putrefaction set in because the fluids had no place to drain.

Doctors eventually solved the problem by connecting the dangling end of the bypassed section to the colon, or to the remaining shortened section of the small intestine. This gave the secretions a place to drain. With certain technical variations, the intestinal bypass is performed this same way today.

The Benefits Intestinal-bypass patients usually lose weight very rapidly during the first few months following the operation. Even if they overeat — and few of them do initially — most of the food passes through their systems without being fully processed. Few patients get down to their ideal weight, but most lose two thirds of their excess fat in the first year and a half following surgery. And for most, the loss is permanent.

The physiological benefits derived from the surgery are the same as benefits from weight loss by any other means. The patient's cardiovascular function improves, and the high blood pressure drops. Insulin response is normalized. The person will have more energy and more mobility, once unburdened of some of the excess weight that may have amounted to one or two hundred pounds or more.

Even if they don't lose all their surplus weight, many bypass patients are more than satisfied to be something approaching a normal size. They like themselves better. They gain confidence and social poise.

Though the operation is filled with serious risks, a high percentage of patients report finding it worthwhile. Some who suffered complications actually chose to die rather than have the operation reversed and risk getting grossly fat again.

The Risks Despite its undeniable capacity to cause weight loss, most surgeons are now reluctant to do intestinal bypasses. The potential hazards are deemed by many to outweigh the benefits. The risks include:

- Liver damage. In some cases, the patient's liver becomes riddled with sacs of pus. No one really knows why they form. The usual explanation is that bacteria in the bypassed loop of the intestine release certain toxins that make their way to the liver, where they begin destroying liver tissue. The body responds by sending white blood cells to the area, which ingest the toxins and then die, forming pus.
- Neurological abnormalities. Nervous system problems may include slurred speech, loss of balance, and disorientation. Again, these side effects are not completely understood, but they are thought to involve toxins released by bacteria in the bypassed intestinal section that can disrupt the chemical transmission of impulses along nerve networks.
- Severe emotional disturbances, including steep mood swings, depression, and confusion. Most bypass patients experience an improved mental outlook as they lose weight rapidly in the months following surgery. But distressing psychological upheavals do afflict a small percentage of the patients. No theory exists to explain these symptoms.
- Chronic, debilitating diarrhea. The food you eat has only two possible fates. It must either be broken down and absorbed for use by your body, or it must be eliminated. The breakdown and absorption take place almost entirely in the small intestine. Since bypass patients have lost the greater part of their small intestines, their ability to break down and absorb food is drastically curtailed. Great amounts of food pass unprocessed through the shortened small intestine and go on to the colon. Water, gas, and excessive waste accumulate rapidly with explosive results. The diarrhea, in turn, can cause dehydration and contribute to vitamin deficiencies and crippling and even fatal mineral deficiencies.
- Irregular heart beats. This symptom is probably caused by the patient's failure to retain enough potassium and other minerals. If you lack potassium, the heart's electrical signals may be disrupted. A serious potassium deficiency can cause death from cardiac arrest.
- Bone softening. Some patients may eventually suffer fractures from stress as mild as mere walking. Presumably, this happens because they are not absorbing enough calcium and phosphorus. Both minerals are essential for strong, healthy bones.
- Anemia, from the failure to absorb enough iron and certain vitamins.
- Shock. Food passes so quickly through the patient's colon that the colon cannot complete its job of reabsorbing minerals. The patient may suffer a salt deficiency that prevents the retaining of enough water, no matter how much is drunk. If this happens, the patient's volume of blood, which is made up mostly of water, may drop so low that the blood no longer exerts much force as it flows through blood vessels. The result is a sudden and severe drop in blood pressure, or shock. Bouts of extreme diarrhea,

with resulting dehydration and shock, can occur days, weeks, months, or even years after the surgery.

- A variety of conditions caused by protein deficiency, including hair loss and cracked nails. This happens because the shortened intestine apparently is not able to absorb enough amino acids to supply hair and nails with adequate protein.
- Every possible vitamin deficiency disease. (Refer to the deficiency diseases on the chart in Chapter 11.) A bypass patient may contract any one of these ailments, or several of them, because of inability to absorb enough vitamins. A follow-up study of bypass patients six years after surgery showed that 76 percent of them were deficient in one or more of the fat-soluble vitamins. Their intestines were not absorbing enough fat, with the result that these vitamins never reached the bloodstream.
- Impaired immunity. Bypass patients are prey to a host of infections. One of my patients who had undergone a bypass had his genitals covered by warts, caused by a virus that his weakened immune system could not fight off. The condition disappeared only after the bypass was reversed. Unfortunately, the cost of the cure was the regaining of this patient's lost weight.
- Bypass enteritis. For some unknown reason, there is a massive bacterial overgrowth in the intestines of some bypass patients. This causes sudden cramping and diarrhea, swelling, and the collecting of fluid in the bypassed loop of the small intestine.
- Kidney stones. With a bypass operation, the chemical environment of the remaining section of small intestine undergoes sweeping changes. Along with not being able to absorb many nutrients one should absorb, the patient may also start absorbing large amounts of food matter one should *not* absorb. For example, *oxalates*, breakdown products of vegetables, normally pass out of the body in a person's stool. But because of some complex chemical changes brought on by the bypass, the patient may begin absorbing a large amount of oxalates into the bloodstream, which must then be eliminated by the kidneys. However, often the oxalates become concentrated in the urine and precipitate out to cause kidney stones.
- Gallstones. When you lose weight quickly, as bypass patients do, fat tissue breaks down rapidly and releases fat into the bloodstream. The result is high blood-fat levels. The liver deals with the situation by clearing fats from the blood as quickly as possible and concentrating them in the bile stored in your gallbladder. The more fat in the bile, the thicker it becomes, and the more likely it is to form gallstones.
- Joint pains. The cause of these pains has not been identified, but it is well established that they tend to occur in bypass patients.

• Pain. Bypass surgery is major surgery, and major surgery almost always involves considerable postoperative pain. The bypass requires an extensive incision in the nerve-rich abdominal wall. Pain will persist until the incision heals. Healing will take six to ten weeks at best, and it may take months. For reasons not entirely understood, obese people heal much more slowly than other people.

Weight Loss with the Bypass Even though the purpose of the bypass is to induce weight loss by limiting intestinal absorption, follow-up studies show that other changes caused by the operation are even more significant.

The most important change is that following the operation, patients usually experience an inexplicable lessening of appetite. The typical bypass patient goes from a high intake of 6,300 calories a day before surgery, to a low of only 1,200 calories a day in the first month or two after the operation. Then intake gradually rises, stabilizing at about 3,500 calories a day by the eighteenth month after surgery and remaining at that level from then on.

In addition, the patients' tastes often change. For instance, studies have shown that following surgery, patients seem to lose much of their taste for sweet food. Again, no one has been able to explain the change. Nor can we account for the fact that eating binges and heavy nighttime eating — common behavior patterns for the morbidly obese — lessen considerably after bypass surgery.

The changes in eating behavior are so significant that scientists estimate that reduced calorie intake accounts for 75 percent of the weight lost by bypass patients. Reduced intestinal absorption accounts for only 25 percent.

But anyone still considering a bypass despite its dangers should also consider this: weight loss from the operation is not unlimited, nor is all of it necessarily permanent. As a rule, patients lose a great deal of weight for several months following surgery. The period of rapid weight loss varies from patient to patient. But very few patients continue to lose for any longer than eighteen months following the operation. After this point, a small percentage of the patients may even begin to regain a few of their lost pounds.

Two factors explain how people with greatly shortened intestines can regain weight. First, their appetites increase so that eventually most of them begin to overeat again, although not to the same degree they did before the operation. Second, the remaining section of intestine becomes more efficient, increasing its absorptive capability to compensate somewhat for the lost intestinal footage. The intestine is able to process some of the excess calories the patients take in, so a little weight may be regained.

By way of compensation, however, the increasing capacity of the intestine means that patients are less prone at this point to suffer the bypass side effects associated with nutritional malabsorption.

STOMACH SURGERY

While the intestinal bypass is on the wane, stomach surgery is on the rise as a treatment for morbid obesity. It has its own set of daunting drawbacks, but most doctors feel that altering the stomach is safer in the long run than tampering with the intestine.

Stomach surgery has nothing to do with the amount of food you can absorb. Its purpose is to limit the amount you eat. This is accomplished by limiting the stomach's capacity to hold food.

The surgery cannot do the job entirely. But stomach surgery can limit how much food you can eat at one sitting. There are patients who circumvent the operation by nibbling small amounts of food virtually around the clock to make up for the big meals they're missing. If they eat too much, however, either they vomit or they risk damaging themselves internally.

You often hear dieters talk of how their stomachs "shrink" after a few days of dieting. Actually, this is not the case. Most dieters do feel fuller on less as they progress with a diet, but no one knows why with any certainty. The most likely reason is that you adapt psychologically to become more satisfied with a restricted intake. In any case, the stomach itself does not change. It never shrinks, nor does it ever stretch. Unless it is surgically altered, its normal capacity of about fifteen to twenty ounces remains the same.

The Procedures There are several different kinds of stomach surgery. Almost all involve closing off a portion of the stomach, either in part or entirely. The capacity the patient retains varies. Surgeons try to tailor it to an individual's needs, making the stomach as small as it needs to be to force weight loss.

The most popular form of stomach surgery currently is stomach stapling. In this procedure, first reported in 1977, staples are inserted in a diagonal line across the stomach. The staples pinch the stomach walls together in a way that divides the stomach into two parts. The upper part may have a capacity as small as two ounces, or even less.

There is a break in the line of staples, leaving a hole about a half-inch in diameter. The hole allows small amounts of food to pass from the top chamber of the stomach into the bottom, and from there on to the intestines to be digested in the normal way.

In a variation on this procedure the stomach is stapled all the way across, leaving no hole for food to pass through. A loop of the small intestine just below the stomach is pulled up and connected to the small upper chamber of the stomach. With this alteration, food passes from the upper chamber directly into the intestine. The loop of intestine remains connected to the lower chamber as well, but only for purposes of drainage. The lower chamber no longer receives any food at all.

Another version of stomach surgery involves partially dividing the stomach surgically instead of with staples. A cut is made most of the way through the stomach toward the top. The edges of the stomach walls are then sutured together along the length of the cut.

What remains is a small upper chamber of the stomach, connected to a larger lower section by a small tube formed by the uncut section. Food then passes from the top to the bottom in much the same way it does with the partial stapling procedure.

Surgical division was the first type of gastric surgery performed, but its use has diminished with the rise of stapling as a slightly less drastic alternative.

The Benefits Most stomach surgery patients lose 55 percent of their extra weight in the first year following surgery. Their diminished size affords them the same physiological, psychological, and social benefits that successful bypass patients enjoy.

Stomach surgery itself is trickier than bypass surgery, mainly because the stomach receives a much richer blood supply than the small intestine does. Bleeding during the operation can be a major problem.

Nevertheless, stomach surgery is safer in the long run than a bypass. Gastric procedures don't cause the severe brain and liver damage that a bypass can inflict. And stomach surgery seldom causes severe mineral imbalances.

The Risks Whether the stomach is stapled or cut, there is a great deal of bleeding during gastric surgery. Sometimes a surgeon cannot control the bleeding locally, on the surface of the stomach itself. He is then forced to tie off a large artery that feeds both the stomach and the nearby spleen, an organ that functions as part of the immune system.

If this is necessary, the spleen has to be removed. Otherwise, it would die anyway from lack of oxygen. It is usually possible for a person to survive quite well without a spleen. But in some patients its absence creates the risk of massive infections from pus-forming bacteria.

A patient who comes through the surgery without mishap still faces some serious postoperative risks:

- Leaking blood. If a patient tries to eat too much after having the surgery, the staples or the stitches that constrict the stomach may tear. This can cause massive, even fatal, hemorrhaging.
- Leaking food and acid. Tearing the staples or stitches can allow food and stomach acid to escape into the abdominal cavity surrounding the stomach. The acid can irritate or even eat through the lining of the cavity, and the food can cause serious, possibly fatal, inflammation of the cavity lining.
- Stomach ulcers. The lower chamber of the stomach is still secreting acid, but it is receiving little or no food to absorb it. As a result, the acid irritates or eats through the stomach lining in some patients. This damage is what constitutes ulcers.
- Swelling. Postsurgical swelling of the stomach can be so bad that the small hole left for the passage of food is swollen shut. The patient has to be fed intravenously until the hole reopens.
- Stomach pain. The patient's remaining stomach capacity may be so small that even the tiniest amount of food can make the stomach feel stretched and painfully full.
- Vomiting. The patient's food may frequently be regurgitated because the stomach is too small to hold it. Vomiting is gastric surgery's most common side effect, afflicting some two thirds of the patients.
- Nutritional deficiencies. Even though the patient is absorbing nutrients normally in the intestines, food intake may be so restricted that one fails to get enough vitamins, minerals, and other nutrients.
- Postoperative pain. As is the case with bypass surgery, gastric surgery is extensive and painful.
- Inadequate weight loss. Some patients are able to sabotage the surgery. Even though they cannot eat much at a single sitting, they can nibble enough high-calorie food over the course of a day to limit their weight loss.

VAGOTOMY

This very recent procedure is novel in its approach, dealing with the nervous system rather than the digestive tract in an attempt to cure morbid obesity.

The *vagus nerve* is really a pair of large nerves running from your brain down the length of your body trunk. They carry impulses to slow the heartbeat and close off certain air tubes in the lungs. From your upper torso, the nerves continue on down to your stomach and intestines.

The vagus nerves carry messages back and forth between the brain and the digestive tract. They help tell you when you're hungry by causing your stomach to begin secreting more digestive acid, your intestines to step up their contractions, and your heart and lungs to slow somewhat. Once you've eaten, the vagus nerves help carry fullness messages back to the brain.

In a vagotomy, the vagus nerves are cut below the diaphragm, the large muscle that divides your upper torso from your belly. Scientists are not sure exactly why, but severing the nerves limits the appetite to the extent that a patient can lose weight fairly easily after the operation.

The procedure does not eliminate hunger and fullness messages entirely, since your body has several other mechanisms for governing those feelings. Nevertheless, a vagotomy produces effects similar to those seen in laboratory animals who lose their appetites after having their hypothalami altered surgically.

The Swedish surgeon J. G. Kral, who first performed the vagotomy, reported in 1978 that his three patients lost significant amounts of weight. A subsequent report from Dr. Kral said that of ten more vagotomy patients, nine lost large amounts of weight easily and without hunger.

The vagotomy is promising in that, so far, no serious side effects have been reported from it. Moreover, in dealing with the nervous system, it mounts an unusually direct attack on the most likely cause of most morbid obesity; that is, a badly malfunctioning hypothalamus.

Nevertheless, it is much too soon to declare the vagotomy universally safe and effective. Too few of the operations have been performed to allow an accurate assessment of immediate ill effects. And since the procedure is so new, there is no way to calculate possible long-range effects.

We do not yet know whether the vagotomy would work for people whose overeating is caused mainly by their response to external cues, but the question may be beside the point. Whether they respond excessively to external cues or not, the morbidly obese appear to overeat mainly in response to genuine hunger signals inflicted on them by faulty hypothalami.

EXOTIC MEASURES FOR THE MERELY PLUMP

The vagotomy is still largely untried. Gastric surgery and the intestinal bypass are very dangerous. Obviously, then, the only people with a legitimate claim even to consider such radical solutions are the morbidly obese.

If your weight problem falls short of morbidity, you should stick to the regimen of exercise, behavior modification, and sensible diet for the surest, safest, and most lasting results. Still, there are people who choose to do otherwise. They look for quicker, easier ways to rid themselves of fat, and some of the "solutions" they come up with are pretty bizarre. Few, if any, produce the desired results over the long haul.

Lipectomy

Outside the realm of surgery for treating morbid obesity, perhaps the most extreme measure used to attack overweight is the *lipectomy*. A lipectomy is also surgery, but it is cosmetic rather than curative. Hardly any surgeon will use this procedure to treat morbid obesity.

A lipectomy is surgery in which the fat itself is cut off the body. It is usually done by a plastic surgeon, who may choose to accept patients more concerned with appearances than with health. In the interest of fashion, people who are by no means grossly fat sometimes seek out this operation.

The fat can be cut away from almost any area or areas the patient designates and the surgeon approves. The fat is removed from beneath the skin. The skin, after slack has been eliminated, is closed over the affected area. The surgery leaves small scars that are usually hidden in some body fold — under the low fold of the belly, for instance, or beneath the buttocks or breasts.

A lipectomy may satisfy vanity for a time, but it's an expensive, painful, and usually temporary way to lose weight. The surgery does remove fat cells contained in the excised fat. However, if the patient overeats afterward, new fat cells will form, and the weight problem will reappear.

I must reiterate here that I do not consider *any* surgery a valid method of dealing with obesity except as a desperate, last-ditch alternative in a case where a patient's life is at risk. Since the lipectomy is not used to treat morbid obesity, I do not think it should be performed at all. It is far too drastic and temporary a remedy for a problem that will respond to less extreme and more permanent conventional treatment.

Drugs

Diet drugs are a multi-million-dollar business in the United States.

Some doctors use prescription appetite suppressants as part of an overall treatment program for their morbidly obese patients.

But many Americans who are only slightly or moderately overweight also use diet drugs — those that can be bought over the counter in almost any drugstore. Very few of these people are helping themselves to permanent weight control. They are merely buying crutches whose dubious benefits don't nearly justify their potential dangers.

STIMULANTS

Most diet drugs are stimulants, and almost all work the same way, by causing your body to produce more of its own natural stimulants, primarily adrenaline and noradrenaline. The artificial stimulants in diet drugs also make you more sensitive to these hormones.

You learned most of what you need to know about adrenaline and noradrenaline in the Hormones section of Chapter 6. You'll remember that both are produced by the adrenal glands near the kidneys and by the nerves. And both are involved in something called the "fight or flee" syndrome.

Adrenaline and noradrenaline levels rise naturally when you experience very strong emotions, such as fear or anger. The hormones alter certain body functions in ways basically intended to help you meet a threat by running or fighting. They speed up your heartbeat and your breathing, for instance, while they depress other body functions not needed for combat or flight.

In this way, adrenaline and noradrenaline are part of your natural defense system. They enable you to react quickly and alertly in the face of danger or stress. Of course, some of us have reached the point in human cultural evolution where we don't necessarily run or do battle in response to strong emotions. We may sit and stew instead. But as you

Drugs that Stimulate Brown Fat

As you know from reading Chapter 6, one of the jobs of the hormone noradrenaline, or norepinephrine, is to stimulate brown fat to generate more heat — and thus burn more calories.

Certain drugs have already been developed that partially block the ability of the central nervous system to use noradrenaline, making more of this hormone available to act as a brown-fat stimulator. If brown-fat activity in overweight people could be increased to the degree enjoyed by those whose brown-fat activity helps make them naturally thin, the benefits would be considerable. Pharmaceutical companies are currently working hard to produce a noradrenaline stimulator potent enough to do this.

Nevertheless, even if this drug becomes available in the future, I would never recommend its use to replace diet and exercise. The side effects can be the same as with other stimulants — nervousness, a rise in blood pressure, constipation, sleeplessness, rapid heartbeat, and, for diabetics, a rise in insulin requirement. For all but the morbidly obese, the only real answer to a weight problem is to change the habits that caused it in the first place, not to take drugs that may have significant negative side effects in the long run.

---

already know, physical evolution lags well behind cultural evolution in many ways. Our bodies, unmindful of our changing ways, still prepare us to react to emotional stress in very basic ways.

One way adrenaline and noradrenaline help do this is by depressing appetite. No one in the grip of rage or panic is ever hungry, since taking time to eat would serve no purpose in such circumstances. So the hormones help direct the digestive tract to slow down and the nervous system to disregard any potential hunger messages.

THE DRAWBACKS OF STIMULANTS

Your body isn't designed to cope with frequent or outsized jolts of hormonal stimulants. Consider, for instance, that at levels ten times the normal, adrenaline can cause panic, irrationality, extreme aggressiveness and hostility, hyperactive mental and physical behavior, hallucinations, and even psychosis. The overstimulation can strain your heart. It can also make you dangerously insensitive to your body's warning signals of pain and fatigue.

Even at only five times normal levels, adrenaline can make you feel jumpy, irritable, and unable to sleep. Some people can tolerate such stimulation better than others, and the amount of artificial stimulants in diet pills is relatively low — in recommended dosage. Even so, diet pills can make a sensitive user nervous, sleepless, and irritable. And the habitual user, even if less sensitive to stimulants, will probably experience bad side effects sooner or later because he or she probably will *not* stick with the recommended dosage.

The problem here is that all stimulants tend to be less effective the more you use them. Scientists call this effect *tachyphylaxis,* from the Greek *tachy,* "quick," and *phylaxis,* "protection." Tachyphylaxis means that your body responds to a foreign substance by reacting against it. But repeated exposure blunts the reaction mechanism, and you become more and more tolerant of the substance.

As tolerance increases, you need the stimulant more often, and in larger amounts, to get the same effect produced by a low dose in the beginning. This is what happens to addicts using such drugs as morphine and heroin, narcotics that must be taken in ever-larger doses to give the user the sought-after effect.

To benefit from stimulants very long, you must eventually start taking them in doses high enough to be dangerous. Therefore, you cannot stay on them indefinitely without endangering your health.

Once you abandon the stimulants, you tend to regain lost weight with depressing speed. Innumerable studies show that while diet pills may help you lose weight faster in the short run, they're useless or downright detrimental for lasting weight control.

Finally, stimulants can be habit-forming. They are not addicting, in that no dire side effects are caused by stopping their use. But you can become psychologically dependent on them, possibly to the point of taking excessive doses to get the effects they produce.

In sum, then, I never recommend the use of stimulants. With prolonged use, dosage high enough to be effective is also high enough to be dangerous. And in the long run, they don't work.

Amphetamines Some stimulants are more dangerous than others. Coffee, for instance, is a stimulant, but drinking four cups a day or less is unlikely to cause any major ill effects for most people.

Amphetamines, on the other hand, are among the strongest stimulants known. They include a variety of synthetic compounds. The familiar trade names are Dexedrine, Benzedrine, and Methedrine. Some college students of the 1950s and 1960s may remember "dexies" and "bennies" as aids in all-night study sessions. It is virtually impossible to sleep after taking one of these drugs until its effects wear off.

Years ago, quite a few doctors prescribed amphetamines for overweight patients. Until tachyphylaxis sets in, the drugs are potent appetite suppressors.

However, they are hardly ever prescribed anymore. The risks they present far outweigh their temporary benefits. Even the healthiest patient is likely to suffer from insomnia and nervousness when on these drugs. Others might experience the whole range of adrenaline-related symptoms. And for patients with bad hearts and certain other infirmities, amphetamines can be deadly.

Phenylpropanolamine Medical knowledge about the dangers of amphetamines has taken them out of circulation almost entirely as diet aids. Yet an amphetaminelike drug is still widely used by dieters. Moreover, you don't even need a prescription to get it. Under many different brand names, it is sold over the counter at most drugstores.

The name of the drug is *phenylpropanolamine*, or *PPA.*

In 1978, an advisory panel to the Food and Drug Administration reviewed some one hundred over-the-counter diet aids. It reported to the FDA that two of them were "safe and effective" for weight loss.

One of the drugs was *benzocaine,* an anesthetic. If you gargle it, it deadens the nerves in your mouth and food doesn't taste good. I'll tell you more about benzocaine later.

The other drug approved by the panel was PPA.

Even though the FDA did not act to accept the panel's findings, the mere suggestion that PPA was safe and effective brought cries of protest from the medical profession and research scientists. Many experts contended that PPA was not effective in the long term and that it could be dangerous in high doses.

Nevertheless, the panel's finding was music to the ears of the diet aids industry. Products containing PPA proliferated rapidly. Many were, and are, widely advertised. Most of the advertising hails the products as "effective" diet aids that "contain no stimulants."

In fact, the average PPA diet pill is about equal in stimulant value to two cups of coffee. This usually isn't enough to hurt you. But neither is it enough to do much to curb your appetite. In higher doses, PPA can dampen your appetite. It is also most certainly a stimulant at such dosage, and it can have amphetaminelike side effects. In other words, to be safe PPA probably won't be very effective, and to be effective it probably won't be entirely safe.

In Australia, where PPA has been available for several years in over-the-counter pills of high dosage, several users have suffered attacks of extremely high blood pressure from taking a single pill. One case of massive brain hemorrhage was attributed to the drug. PPA has also been known to aggravate heart disease and diabetes.

I would no more recommend that a patient take PPA than I would prescribe amphetamines. I do not believe the drug is safe, nor is it effective for lasting weight control. It is also possible for a patient to become dependent on PPA, just as on amphetamines.

NICOTINE

One can only guess how many smokers would like to kick the habit, but are inhibited by a fear of gaining weight. The fear is by no means unfounded. You do risk weight gain when you stop smoking, both for physical and psychological reasons.

Nicotine, the addicting substance in tobacco, is a stimulant. Like any other stimulant, it acts on your central nervous system to suppress your appetite. Consequently, an almost universal symptom of nicotine withdrawal is a greatly increased appetite. Along with this, the person trying to quit smoking must cope with the loss of a habitual form of oral gratification, puffing on a cigarette. The frequent temptation is to replace this with another form of oral gratification, eating.

Certainly, the smokers among you will have to muster everything you know about behavior modification, diet, and exercise if you're to avoid gaining weight during the difficult period of withdrawal from nicotine. Nevertheless, I strongly recommend that you tackle the problem and try to quit — and not only because of the many obvious health hazards posed by smoking.

I've told you time and again that exercise is crucial to long-term weight control. Very few smokers are able to exercise effectively, since their hearts and lungs don't function as well as those of nonsmokers.

There are several good organizations that can help you ward off weight gain while you ditch your cigarettes. I suggest you seek out such a group if you have tried and failed in the past to quit smoking, or to quit without gaining weight.

BENZOCAINE

I agree with the FDA advisory panel that benzocaine is safe. No important side effects have been reported from its use.

Nevertheless, its "effectiveness" is very much in doubt. People who lack the will to diet effectively without benzocaine can hardly be expected to put up with the drug indefinitely either. It tastes bad, creates numbness in the mouth, and removes most of the taste from all food, not just fattening food. It can discourage a worthwhile effort to learn good eating habits, and it is never an adequate substitute for those habits.

THYROID HORMONES AND DIGITALIS

Thyroid hormones are the same chemicals that your thyroid gland makes for you. You'll remember from Chapter 6 that they are antifat hormones that heighten metabolism. When administered as medication they are either synthesized in a laboratory or taken from the glands of animals.

Giving thyroid hormones to someone with a normal thyroid gland is a terrible practice. At doses equal to what your body produces on its own, they are completely ineffective for weight loss. To speed up your metabolism, the dosage must be more than three times as high. At such dosage, they can cause rapid or irregular heartbeats and high blood pressure. They can be fatal, particularly if taken in combination with other stimulants or with diuretics or with heart medicines such as digitalis.

Digitalis is a heart drug that may be prescribed in conjunction with thyroid hormones. The digitalis slows the rapid heartbeat the hormones can cause. But the digitalis itself can cause nausea and vomiting.

There are a few doctors who prescribe these substances for their obese patients, but I mention this practice only to condemn it. It can kill you.

FENFLURAMINE

I never recommend drugs for weight loss. But it must be said in its behalf that *fenfluramine* (brand name Pondimin) is the least objectionable of the drugs used to suppress appetite.

Fenfluramine's chemical structure is similar to that of amphetamines, but the drug is not a stimulant. It is, in fact, a depressant that tends to make you feel tired.

Fenfluramine is thought to act by making your body more responsive to serotonin. Serotonin is the brain hormone you learned about in Chapter 7, the one believed to be a natural appetite suppressant.

Like virtually all drugs, fenfluramine is tachyphylactic. It may also induce dependence after a patient takes it over a period of time. However, some researchers have found that these problems can be solved to an extent by administering the drug in intervals. The patient might take it for a week, go without it for a week, then resume it for a week, and so on.

But fenfluramine should be administered, if at all, only under the constant care of a doctor. In some people, it can cause high blood pressure, glaucoma, drowsiness, diarrhea, and dryness of the mouth.

And I raise the same objection to this drug that I do to all weight-control drugs. Obesity is a long-range problem that requires long-range solutions — not temporary crutches. Most physicians are unlikely to recommend that you stay on fenfluramine for a lifetime. Depending on any drug can undermine your will to make the permanent changes in eating behavior and activity patterns that you need for permanent weight loss.

SPIRULINA

If you ever saw blue-green scum on a stagnant pond, you saw the raw material for *spirulina,* a product made from algae. Since it contains protein, spirulina is sold as a food, not a drug. Nevertheless, it is supposed to have druglike properties for killing your appetite, so it deserves mention here.

A while back, the *National Enquirer* — a dubious source of medical information — reported that spirulina contains the amino acid *phenyl-alanine,* which "acts on your brain's appetite center to switch off your hunger pangs. So you can eat less — and lose weight."

It's hard to imagine how the newspaper reached this conclusion. There is no known medical research that even suggests that phenylalanine has any effect whatever on appetite. Just possibly, the report got its amino acids confused. There is an amino acid, *tryptophan,* that's needed for the formation of serotonin. And serotonin, as you know, is believed to be a natural appetite inhibitor.

This does not mean that I recommend you load yourself with tryptophan to kill your appetite. Taking supplements of it won't do anything for you unless you are deficient in this particular amino acid. And hardly anyone is, since the average American diet is full of it. Milk and poultry, for instance, are loaded with tryptophan.

But I don't recommend that you try to spirulina either. The *National Enquirer* article was followed by booming spirulina sales, and it continues to be popular. It also continues to be worthless for weight loss, as far as medical science can determine.

STARCH BLOCKERS

Starch blockers are another weight-loss fad that never should have happened. It is highly questionable whether the starch blockers work at all. And if they do work, they may not be safe for all users.

In scores of variations from different manufacturers, starch blockers burst on the commercial diet scene early in the summer of 1982. Usually sold in capsule form, the blockers were supposed to let you pig out on pasta, potatoes, and other tasty starches at a drastically reduced cost in calories.

The theory behind the starch blockers goes like this: a group of enzymes called *amylases* are found in your saliva and your intestinal juices. Their job is to break down starch into single sugars that your body can absorb. If the amylases are prevented from doing their job, the starch cannot be digested properly, and must pass on through your system without releasing calories. Some starch-blocker proponents claim their product can eliminate as many as 400 starch calories from any given meal.

The theory sounds good, but reliable research has punched some holes in it. Studies in Germany showed that starch blockers slowed the action of amylases but did not stop it. This means that while you might absorb calories from starches at a slower rate while taking the blockers, you would nevertheless absorb most, if not all of them, eventually. These same studies showed that starch blockers had no effect on starch in cooked foods.

A study at the University of California at Davis showed that starch blockers failed to prevent weight gain in rats. Rodents aside, research at Pima Community College in Tucson, Arizona, showed that starch blockers should not work in humans either. The Tucson study demonstrated that starch blockers work only within a narrow range of acid-alkaline balance, and that the human stomach is far too acid to fall within that range.

Dr. J. John Marshall, a chemist at Notre Dame University, originated the concept of starch blockers. He isolated a chemical from kidney beans and soybeans that partially blocked amylases in the test tube. Dr. Marshall contends his discovery has produced remarkable results in human weight loss.

So far, however, those results have not been duplicated by other researchers. I should also note that starch-blocker manufacturers have not always been as scrupulous in their methods as Dr. Marshall was. Rather than extracting any chemicals from soybeans or kidney beans, some producers reportedly have merely ground up the beans themselves and marketed this worthless substance as a starch blocker.

The best evidence that some starch blockers may work is also a good argument against their use. Some people who take the blockers experience explosive flatulence and diarrhea — presumably an indication that starch is not being digested. An absence of this unpleasant and embarrassing side effect is also an indication that the supposed starch blocker is not doing the job.

Doctors were quick to warn diabetics away from starch blockers, which may tamper with blood-sugar levels. And there has been no extended research to prove conclusively that starch blockers are safe for the general public. Tampering with enzymes is, after all, an interference with the body's normal operation, and it shouldn't be undertaken lightly.

At the time this book was being published, the debate over the efficacy and safety of starch blockers had landed in the lap of the federal Food and Drug Administration, which has moved to have the substances taken off the market.

Other Methods

Lipectomies and drugs are not the only exotic measures around. Several offbeat weight-loss methods have seen vogues and declines in America in recent years, and some enjoy continuing public favor. Some are more or less humorous, but all are of doubtful value.

ACUPUNCTURE

While dining in a restaurant one evening in 1980, I found myself staring at a stout man engaged in a strange ritual. Each time the pastry cart rolled by him, he stared at it hungrily and began pulling madly on his left ear.

I didn't know what to make of this until several weeks later when I heard about acupuncture and ear stapling for weight loss.

Acupuncture is the ancient Chinese art of inserting needles at special points on the body to relieve pain. Its enthusiasts include some American weight-loss gurus, who allege that acupuncture can affect some feeding center in the brain. This center is supposed to be located somewhere near the ear.

On the basis of this thesis, some people had staples placed at certain sites on their ears. Fondling these staples was supposed to allay hunger when temptation threatened.

People with stapled ears were certainly interesting to watch, but there is no evidence that the technique worked. The best scientists in the obesity field still don't know all there is to know about how appetite works, and one could hardly expect the staple vendors to know more.

In any case, ear stapling is no longer very popular.

JAW WIRING

To eat solid food you have to chew, and to chew you have to move your jaws. If you can't move your jaws, you're very likely to lose weight.

This perfectly rational line of thought has led some obese people to have their jaws wired together. *Mandibular fixation* is the technical name for this measure.

Patients who have their jaws wired shut can ingest only liquids. Usually, they subsist largely on liquid protein preparations, perhaps supplemented with other nutrients. These patients almost always lose weight, and they do it fast.

But there are problems.

You can't brush your teeth properly or floss them with your jaws wired, so dental problems are a virtual certainty after a time. In addition, the jaw muscles tend to atrophy, or weaken from disuse, so the wires must come off sooner or later. Once they are removed, most patients must learn to chew all over again. But they quickly master this skill. And when they do, they usually regain their lost weight and arrive back where they started.

If all this doesn't discourage you from getting wired up, consider the pain. Jaw wiring is a surgical procedure, and it usually hurts.

HYPNOSIS

If you can't get your conscious mind to diet effectively, give your subconscious a whack at it. This is the idea behind hypnosis for weight control.

The hypnosis patient is put into a trance by a doctor, a reputable hypnotist, or, sometimes, a quack. Once the trance state is induced, the patient's subconscious gets helpful suggestions: "You love celery and zucchini. You hate pizza and ice cream. You like small meals. Overeating is revolting."

Hypnosis does help some people to lose weight for periods ranging from a few weeks to a few months. But studies show that hypnosis has one of the highest recidivism rates of any weight-loss method. This means that people who opt for hypnosis are among the likeliest of all weight-watchers to regain whatever they lose.

The follow-up studies indicate that hypnosis is usually ineffective in altering a person's dietary inclinations and activity patterns permanently, no matter how well it works in the early stages. It appears that sustained *conscious* effort of the sort encouraged by behavior modification is what's needed to make you change the grain of deeply entrenched tastes.

NEGATIVE BIOFEEDBACK

The central notion of negative biofeedback is that if rewards won't help you toward good eating habits, punishment might.

Negative biofeedback treatments set up a system of extreme negative reinforcement that is supposed to make you associate food with unpleasantness.

There are clinics throughout much of the country that specialize in this approach. A typical negative biofeedback treatment goes something like this: You are told to think about food. When you do, you're given a mild electric shock. The procedure is repeated again and again until the technician doing it is satisfied that you are sufficiently conditioned.

Negative biofeedback may appeal to the self-punitive natures of some chronic weight-watchers, but the success of its tactics is very much in doubt.

The overwhelming majority of psychologists and obesity specialists believe that negative reinforcement is far inferior to positive reinforcement in altering human behavior.

As tyrants have learned for centuries, people respond to pain or fear only as long as they have to. Their every instinct tells them to remove the source of the pain and fear in the most direct way possible. In the case of negative biofeedback, the patient is far more likely to remove the source of discomfort not by altering bad habits, but by abandoning the unpleasant treatments. Even if one stays with the method for the prescribed course of treatment, the new "conditioning" is seldom if ever permanent. It usually does not survive very long once the immediate source of discomfort — the electric shock — ceases to be a threat.

On the other hand, people respond to pleasure because they want to — not because they have to — and they are therefore likely to continue responding indefinitely. This is why positive reinforcement in the form of praise and rewards is a basic element of behavior modification.

Responsible behavior modification programs such as those used by reputable weight-loss clinics and organizations never use negative reinforcement.

Negative biofeedback has never been shown to have significant lasting value for weight control. Positive reinforcement has proved itself to be quite effective. The obvious moral here is that your chances of success are much greater if you work with human nature instead of against it.

HOPE FOR THE FUTURE?

There are smokers who won't quit smoking because they believe that medical science will soon come up with easy cures for emphysema, bronchitis, and lung cancer. Similarly, there are fat people who won't exercise and eat right because they're sure some wonderful fat cure is just around the corner.

Don't hold your breath. It is possible that someday, medical research will produce a biochemical cure for obesity. But it's not likely that many of us will live to see it. If you don't believe that, consider the state of some current obesity research.

Antiabsorptives

Every dieter's dream is to eat anything and everything you want and still lose weight. That is exactly the promise held out by the search for chemicals that might keep you from absorbing food.

Scientists have already come up with a substance called *cholestyramine* (brand name Questran). It is sometimes used to help reduce cholesterol levels. Cholestyramine binds to cholesterol in the intestinal tract to keep it from entering the bloodstream.

But cholestyramine was never intended as an antiobesity drug, and it is a far cry from being a safe and effective all-purpose antiabsorptive agent. It can interfere with fat absorption and prevent your body from absorbing fat-soluble vitamins. You learned from the chart in Chapter 11 what deficiencies in these vitamins can mean. Cholestyramine can also cause severe constipation and headaches.

The search goes on for a substance that will limit the absorption of all calorie-bearing nutrients and still be safe.

There are occasional reports — usually in the popular press rather than in medical journals — about some chemical that's supposed to prevent the physical absorption of calories. But no such substance has undergone substantial testing to prove its value or its safety.

Even if such a substance were available, it would have to be administered with extreme care, under a physician's careful supervision. When you're not absorbing calories, you're not absorbing nutrients either. Taking a complete antiabsorptive could produce all the nutrition deficiency side effects of the bypass operation, and more.

I find it unimaginable that a total antiabsorptive, or anything even approaching it, will ever be available over the counter. And I believe it will be years before doctors will be prescribing antiabsorptives for weight loss. If ever. A person taking one indiscriminantly could become sick in a staggering number of ways; could die from problems caused by mineral imbalances or vitamin deficiencies; or could simply die from starvation, even while gorging.

Stomach Ballooning

One of the best things you can say about antiabsorptives is that they look pretty good compared with another novel method being proposed — stomach ballooning.

For this one, you need a ten-cent balloon attached to a long tube. You swallow the balloon, thread the tube out through your nose, and tape it in place. Then you fill the balloon with water and air, so that it fills about half your stomach. Next, eat all you want. You won't have room for much.

This doesn't strike me as much of a breakthrough. At best, it might be some sort of temporary answer for morbidly obese people who want some of the benefits of gastric surgery without the surgery itself.

But stomach surgery is usually permanent. For lasting benefits, the balloon routine presumably would have to be done several times a day for the rest of your life. Imagine having to visit a doctor before every meal. Worse, imagine sitting at your kitchen table swallowing balloons and threading tubes through your nose.

The balloon technique was pioneered in Canada a few years ago. To my knowledge, no doctor in the United States is using it.

THE LAST WORD

The morbidly obese may truly have no choice but to try to save their lives with painful, hazardous surgery. But what about the rest of you?

Is it really easier to swallow balloons or have your jaws wired together than to eat properly? Does it make more sense to have fat cut off your body or to tamper with dangerous or useless drugs than it does to exercise? And what possible reason is there to punish yourself with electric shock or tamper with your subconscious through hypnosis when you could try behavior modification instead?

Exercise, proper eating, and behavior modification may strike you as daunting at first. But if you haven't given them a full and fair chance, you haven't experienced the great benefits they offer — not just in weight loss, but in all-around mental and physical well-being.

And like them or not, exercise, diet, and behavior modification are the best answers we have for the problem of fat. They may be the best we'll ever have.

There are no shortcuts to slenderness. There are no substitutes for your own desire and motivation, applied to the tried and true methods. But those methods do work. And because they work, you never have to be fat.

Finally, it's your choice.

19.

STAYING THIN

If this book has done its job, finishing it should not be an ending for you, but a beginning.

It should start you on a rational road toward a slimmer, healthier, more vigorous, and more satisfying life. It should keep you to the high ground of good nutrition and proper exercise, and away from the blind alleys of dangerous fad diets and worthless gimmicks.

I have promised you no miracles and offered no easy ways for getting thin because there are none. There are only the facts — facts that are often complicated, seldom glamorous, and sometimes hard to face. *But learning those facts, as you have done, is the single most important step you'll ever take toward ending your weight problem, finally and forever.*

WHAT HAVE YOU LEARNED?

Here are some of the more important facts that I hope you'll take with you:

1. There is nothing intrinsically bad about body fat. A certain amount of fat is necessary to our very survival, and the ability to store fat was one of mankind's great evolutionary coups. Fat is bad only when there's too much of it. "Too much" is defined as more fat than 10 percent above the ideal body-fat percentages of 15 percent for men and 25 percent for women.

2. Fat is not innately ugly any more than it's intrinsically bad. A cultural preference for slenderness or fatness is merely a matter of fashion. Fashions are shaped largely by socioeconomic conditions and cultural heritage, and they're always subject to change.

3. We live in a society that is schizoid about fat. We value slenderness

probably more than any other culture in history ever has. Yet as many as 40 percent of all Americans are overweight. In trying to bridge the gulf between the cultural ideal of beauty and the reality of excess pound-age, many people have become desperate in their effort to lose weight. The desperation has sometimes made them easy prey to much outra-geous hokum surrounding the subject of fat.

4. A particularly pernicious bit of nonsense is the idea that your worth as a person depends on the size of your body. Diet evangelists would have you believe that fat people are either weak-willed moral defectives who revel in gluttony, or psychological defectives victimized by their own appetites. In fact, there is no evidence that the obese are different from anyone else in terms of moral fitness or psychological stability. Obesity is an extremely complex problem with diverse causes, no pat solutions, and with many mysteries still unplumbed.

5. We should regard obesity not at all as a moral problem, and only parenthetically as a cosmetic problem. It is most truly a medical problem. You can be as much as 10 percent above your ideal body-fat level without endangering your health. But beyond that, you put yourself in jeopardy. Obesity is associated with a host of ailments, not the least of which are cardiovascular diseases. It can impair the quality of your life, and it can shorten your life span.

6. Not all people are equal in the race to be thin. Some inherit the tendency to be fat, and some inherit fattening habits that become in-grained in their eating behavior and activity patterns. Some people are more sluggish than others metabolically. Some have less efficient internal controls for regulating appetite. Women have built-in handicaps result-ing mostly from their reproductive role.

7. Whatever the inequities, you are *never* fated to be fat. Bad habits can be changed with behavior modification techniques that aim at making permanent changes in your lifestyle. Slow metabolisms and faulty ap-pestats can be tuned up and normalized with exercise.

8. The one and only way to lose weight is to expend more calories than you take in. Limiting calories is important for weight loss. But in your zeal to get slim, you must never sacrifice proper nutrition. You can lose weight safely only with a balanced diet — one that provides all the necessary carbohydrates, protein, fat, vitamins, and minerals. Resist the lure of nutritionally unsound fad diets. They seldom, if ever, afford you permanent weight loss. And they can seriously impair your health.

9. Diet without exercise is the weight-watcher's recipe for failure. You

may lose weight with diet alone, but your chances of keeping it off permanently are practically infinitesimal. You're merely setting yourself up for the dangerous and depressing yo-yo syndrome of quick loss and quick gain, which will probably leave you fatter than before.

10. Exercise is the single most important factor in achieving permanent weight control. Given our evolutionary legacy, inactivity is the signal for our bodies to store fat. Vigorous movement is the signal to expend calories at a high rate. Proper exercise promotes the kind of metabolic activity that helps keep you thin. It also helps you control your eating — not with unnatural self-deprivation, but with a naturally diminished appetite. Aerobic exercise intense enough to raise your pulse to 120 beats a minute for thirty minutes three times a week is essential for healthy, lasting weight loss. If you combine this kind of exercise with sensible eating and behavior modification, there's no reason why you can't be thin, fit, and healthy for life.

WHERE DO YOU GO FROM HERE?

Forward. Starting now.

Telephone your doctor *today* and schedule a checkup. Plan in advance to discuss the diet and exercise you want to undertake. This will help the doctor cover all the bases in determining any restrictions you may need to observe. Make a list of questions to ask, including an inquiry about a stress test. Ask about your blood pressure. Ask the doctor to help you gauge your body-fat percentage, or to direct you to someone who can. Ask anything you feel you need to know about your body. The right doctor will be interested enough in the healthy lifestyle you're trying to adopt to answer all your questions.

Next on your agenda for today: construct the food diary that will serve as the basis for your behavior modification program. Go back and scan the behavior modification chapter in this book (Chapter 14) for specific tips. Add to it with a list of ideas you think may be of specific help to you.

Also for today: make a list of the foods you need for the Getting Thin Diet. Go to the supermarket and buy them. Start the diet. Now.

BACKSLIDING

Sometimes a weight-watcher's worst enemy is one's own yen for perfection, coupled with a strong proclivity for guilt.

You may have held to your diet wonderfully for several days, but when you yield to temptation and have a pat of butter, all is lost! You may be progressing nicely with your exercise program. But an unexpected emergency at the office makes you miss a workout, and lo, catastrophe! You messed up. You blew it. You couldn't do it right, so you might as well not bother at all. You might as well eat. You might as well sit around and do nothing.

Please, please avoid this senseless, destructive trap. It's harmful in itself because guilt is a dead weight that saps your motivation and confidence. And it's harmful in what it shows about the way you're thinking. It indicates that you're driving intensely toward some short-term goal, when instead you should be thinking in terms of a lifelong project that is bound to have its ups and downs.

You're not just trying to change your weight, you're trying to change your whole way of life. This is a very tall order. It requires not just willpower and drive, but patience, persistence, and a reasonable amount of compassion for yourself.

Of course you will lapse. Expect to. You're human. There is no disgrace in lapsing; the disgrace lies in letting the lapses get the better of you so that you quit trying.

Prepare for lapses. Realize they're going to come, and keep them in perspective. Always remember that your commitment to a healthy, active lifestyle and good eating habits can be renewed at any time. Backsliding never means that you're lost beyond redemption.

The lapses will be easier to handle if they're not prolonged. The sooner you get back on your program, the better off you are. A short lapse is less demoralizing than a long one. A short one means losing less ground. And a quick return to your regimen will help reinforce your commitment to your long-term goals.

If you've gone off your diet, your first step in getting back on is to resume your food diary. Remember, being aware of what you eat contributes to the feeling that you're in control of your food intake. Don't try to "atone" for your misstep by starving yourself after a lapse. Just return to the sensible eating outlined in your diet.

If you've lapsed in regard to exercise, the remedy will depend mostly on the length of the lapse. Remember the rule of reversibility: once you stop exercising, the endurance that's so vital to aerobic workouts deserts you very fast. You can lose your stamina in only two weeks or so. If this happens, you must go back to the beginning and start working up once more to your final goal of three thirty-minute workouts a week. It may sound tedious. But if you did it before, you can do it again, and it may be easier this time with your previous experience under your belt.

GETTING TO KNOW YOUR "NEW SELF"

Expecting too much of yourself is the most common and obvious pitfall a weight-watcher faces. But there's another, more subtle trap that you should be aware of: the difficulty some people encounter in coping with success.

Sometimes former fatties who have slimmed down feel that they have become a "new self" in a literal and somewhat disturbing way. They look in the mirror, see a slender body, and say, "That really isn't me." The new image may be so disquieting and unfamiliar that, consciously or not, the person sets about to erase it by regaining weight.

Forewarned is forearmed. If you anticipate this image problem, you can take steps from the outset of your program to guard against it. As you lose weight gradually, stay in touch with what's happening to your body. Look at yourself often and become thoroughly familiar with the changes taking place. If you find yourself slipping back into fattening habits after you've reached your goal, take a careful, honest look at your motives. If you feel you need some professional help in this endeavor, get it. A psychiatrist or psychologist may not be called for. Counselors for good weight-control programs are familiar with the problem, and can advise members on how to handle it.

TOMORROW AND FOREVER

Your doctor's appointment is made. Your food diary is at hand. The diet has begun. You're on your way.

The last, best advice I can give you is this: muster enthusiasm for the adventure you're beginning. Enthusiasm should be easy. You have much to look forward to.

You're going to feel stronger, more energetic, more relaxed, more alive. You're going to have a sense of well-being, of optimism, of control over your life.

You're going to look better. You're going to feel more confident. You're going to enjoy shopping for clothes, and you'll wear them with pride. You may find yourself more eager to get out in the world, to see people, to take up activities and projects you may never have considered before.

When you're happier with yourself, you'll probably find that you become happier with others. It's easy to feel antagonism toward a world in which you feel you don't quite fit. A sense of exclusion and isolation is not uncommon among overweight people in our thin-oriented age. Losing weight can help free you from the cocoon of your own self-consciousness so you can be more caring, more giving to others.

A new self? You may think of it that way. But perhaps it's truer to say that starting now, you're setting out to make the self you are everything that it was meant to be.

INDEX

Accidents, 28, 34
Acupuncture, 280–281
Additive diets, 144–145, 146–148, 158
Adenosine triphosphate (ATP), 59
Adler, Bill, 155
Adolescents, 80, 82, 103, 104, 105–106
Adrenal glands, 55, 65, 71. *See also* Adrenaline; Noradrenaline
Adrenaline: and fat, 65; and appetite, 71–72, 75–76; and diet drugs, 272–273, 275
Aerobic exercise, 211, 216, 220, 233, 254, 288, 290. *See also* Exercise
Africa, 12, 13
Age: and energy vs. calories, 211; and exercise, 215, 221, 232–239
Alcoholic beverages, 177–178, 193, 194, 195, 244
Alexeev, Vasily, 36
Amino acids: and diet drugs, 278; and exercise, 204; and fad diets, 145, 148, 149, 153; as nutrients, 109, 163; and obesity surgery, 265; and protein, 120–123. *See also* Protein
Ammonia, 122, 152
Amphetamines, 274–275, 276, 277
Amylases, 279–280
Anabolic hormone, 90
Androgens, 94
Anemia, 264
Annual Review of Medicine, 99
Anorexia nervosa, 103–104, 105, 258
Antiabsorptives, 283–284
Appestat, 69, 73, 74, 77–78, 161, 211, 260, 287. *See also* Appetite
Appetite: and acupuncture, 281; and anorexia, 105; and diet drugs, 272, 273, 275, 276, 277, 278; and eating habits, 194, 195, 196; and exercise, 6, 68, 72–73, 75, 77–78, 202, 203; and externality theory, 76–

77; and fad diets, 142–143, 151, 158; and morbid obesity, 259; and obesity surgery, 262, 266, 270–271; and pregnancy, 90, 92; and theories of hunger, 62, 68–73, 91; and theories of satiety, 73–76; and worthless workouts, 248, 249. *See also* Appestat
Arteries, 33; and brown fat, 53–54; and cardiovascular disease, 29–30, 50, 127, 135, 152; and exercise, 205; and fad diets, 144; and vitamins, 132. *See also* Bloodstream; Hardening of arteries
Arthritis, 28, 30, 31
Artificial sweeteners, 139, 176, 177, 178, 179, 180
Ascorbic acid, 131. *See also* Vitamin C
Asia, 13
Athletes: body-fat percentages of, 40; and calorie burnoff, 51; and exercise, 212, 217, 221, 228, 245; and menstruation, 88; women as, 93
Atkins, Robert, 141–143, 146; Diet Revolution, 141–143, 151, 152
Australia, 276

Baboons, 73
Back and shoulders stretching routine, 224
Backaches, 95
Backsliding, 289–290
Bacteria, 115, 117, 263, 264, 265, 269
Balanchine, George, 11
Banting, William, 141
Basal metabolism, 51
Bears, 19, 23, 51, 52
Beauty: fat and economics of, 13–16; fat, thinness, and, 8–11, 12, 286; and self-image, 17–18, 102–103
"Behavioral Control of Overeating," 188

Weight loss (*cont.*)
151, 157, 158; and fat cells, 83, 86; and
Getting Thin Diet, 160–161, 162, 176,
181, 182; and guilt, 106; and hormones,
61, 63, 65, 66; importance of, 287; industry, 3, 17; and merely plump, 271–
283; and morbid obesity, 258–271; and
pregnancy, 24, 92, 93; and worthless
workouts, 248, 253, 254; and yellow fat,
53. *See also* Dieting; Diets; Fad diets
Weight Watchers, 199
Winnick, Myron, 139
Woman Doctor's Diet for Women, 151
Women: body-fat percentages, 40–41, 42,
44, 46, 87, 88, 286; energy needs and
calories, 110, 206–210; and fad diets, 143,
150; fat and emotions, 102–103; hormones, 66, 87–91; as fatter sex, 17, 87–
94, 287; and Getting Thin Diet, 183, 184;
health problems of, 28, 30, 31–32, 81,

93–96; minerals for, 134; morbid obesity,
259; prejudice toward fat, 99–100, 103–
106; and sexuality, 96–97; social attitudes
toward fat, 4, 8–12, 14–15; and strength
training, 254; and weight charts, 36, 37–
39. *See also* Menstruation; Pregnancy
Women's movements, 12, 104–105
Working, 193–194, 206–207, 209–210
Workout: in exercise, 220–222, 227, 231–
247; worthless, 248–257

Yalow, Rosalyn, 74
Yellow fat, 53, 54, 59, 90
Yoga, 199
Yo-yo syndrome, 5, 6, 49, 50, 86, 110,
151, 155, 156, 157, 162, 187, 200, 203,
288

Zen Macrobiotic Diet, 155–156
Zinc, 113, 133